Body therapy

AND FACIAL WORK

Body therapy
AND FACIAL WORK

Mo Rosser

Hodder & Stoughton

A MEMBER OF THE HODDER HEADLINE GROUP

DEDICATION

To Gwyn, Jeff and Sue.
With thanks for their constant help and support

British Library Cataloguing in Publication Data

Rosser, Mo
  Body Therapy and Facial Work: Electrical
  Treatments for Beauty Therapists
  I. Title
  646.7

ISBN 0–340–58511–0

First published 1994
Impression number 10 9 8 7 6 5 4 3 2 1
Year   1998 1997 1996 1995 1994

Typeset by Wearset, Boldon, Tyne and Wear.
Printed in Great Britain for Hodder & Stoughton Educational, a division of Hodder Headline Plc, Mill Road, Dunton Green, Sevenoaks, Kent TN13 2YA by Thomson Litho Limited.

Contents

Acknowledgments

I am indebted to the following for their help and advice during the preparation of this book: Greta Couldridge, Northampton College, for meticulously reading and advising on all aspects of the text, and Lyn Goldberg, Kay Judd and Karen Denison of the London College of Fashion for reading and advising on sections of the text.

To the following for specialist advice: Dr Rosemary J. S. Jones, Senior Research fellow, Bristol University (Chapter 5). Mr J. Hawk, Consultant Dermatologist, St Thomas's Hospital, London (Chapter 7) and Vanessa Puttnick, Technical Director, The Hairdressing and Beauty Equipment Centre, London N7 for technical advice. Thanks also to Jorge Centofanti, Marketing Director, Ultratone, London W1H for reading and advice on Chapter 6.

Thank you to the following companies for supplying and allowing us to reproduce photographs: The Hairdressing and Beauty Equipment Centre, 262 Holloway Road, London N7; Ultratone, 36 George Street, London W1H; Trimtone Ltd, Clacton Road, London N17; Bretherton Therapy Products, 29 Orchard Road, Beeston; Taylor Reeson, Commerce Way, Lancing, West Sussex; Cathiodermie, René Guinot, The Clock House, Ascot, Berkshire; Depilex, 2 Marsh Lane, Nantwich, Cheshire; Thalgo, Thalgo House, Blackheath Village, London SE3.

Finally, thanks to the following for typing services: Diane McIntier, and Sheila Jarvis, and Suzie Robertson for preparation of the manuscript. The commissioned photographs were taken by Roddy Paine and Jonathan Marsh.

Lastly many thanks to beauty therapists Linda Le Mesurier and Jennifer Jayarajan and to students Dawn Love, Sylvia Camancho, Emma Sloly, Lucy Marshal, Claire Davey and Antonia Burrell, for modelling for the photographs in this book.

Introduction: The care and comfort of the client

Although it is recognised that both male and female clients frequent salons, this text refers to the female throughout for simplicity.

Before any treatment can commence the client must be placed in a comfortable well supported position.

The care and comfort of the client throughout the treatment is extremely important.

Clients derive the greatest benefit from any treatments if they are helped to relax and made to feel cosseted and well cared for. Good rapport with the client is essential to gain her confidence and the friendliness and competence of the therapist will ensure that she returns for further treatments.

Always greet the client in a friendly courteous and smiling manner. Call her by her name as this creates an instant feeling of security. The surname can be used at first progressing to christian names as rapport develops.

Remember that first impressions are important.

Conduct the client to the working area or cubicle. Ask her to undress and give her a robe or large towel to wear. Give her a pair of disposable slippers or place a sheet of clean paper on the floor for her to stand on.

Sit down with the client for the consultation. Be prepared to discuss the various suitable treatments with the client and give her appropriate advice. Should the client request an unsuitable treatment, dissuade her gently giving reasons why the treatment would not be appropriate and offer an alternative and more effective treatment.

After full consultation the treatment should commence.

Facial treatments usually commence with a cleanse and tone.

Body treatments commence with a shower and some form of pre-heating.

Prone lying

Supine lying

Recovery position

Positioning the client on the bed or couch.

- The bed should be prepared in advance.
- Cover with a clean towel or fitted cover.
- Cover pillows with a clean towel.
- Cover the bed and pillows with disposable paper sheet, ie bed roll.
- Two towels should be provided to cover the client. Blankets may be used over the towel if the client feels cold, however they are difficult to launder and should not come in contact with the client.
- A supply of extra pillows and towels should be available for extra support when necessary.

The position of the client will depend on the treatment. Clients may be placed

Prone lying (face down)

Supine lying (face up) or half lying, ie back raised at an angle.

Recovery position ie side lying with under arm and leg behind and upper arm and leg bent to support the body.

In the prone position it is more comfortable for the client if the feet project over the edge of the bed. This prevents stretching of the ligaments at the front of the ankle. The head may be turned to one side. A pillow under the abdomen may be more comfortable and will round out a hollow back.

In the supine or half lying position a pillow to support the head will improve comfort. A pillow under the knees and thighs will also improve comfort and aid relaxation.

In the recovery position a pillow under the head and a pillow supporting the upper leg improve comfort.

Always ensure that the treatment room/area

- is warm, but well ventilated without draughts;
- is private, quiet and relaxing;
- is hygienic, very clean and tidy;
- has soft, subdued lighting, with good lighting available when needed;
- has all necessary commodities neatly arranged, and the couch and trolley scrupulously clean.

For salon and personal hygiene see pages 216–218.

CHAPTER 1 *Basic science*

Figure 1.1   *High frequency and galvanic portable unit*

OBJECTIVES

After you have studied this chapter you will be able to:

1 List the three states of matter.
2 Differentiate between an element and a compound.
3 Describe the structure of an atom.
4 Discuss the formation of *ions* and explain the terms *cation* and *anion*.
5 Describe the flow of electrons through a conductor.
6 Differentiate between conductors and non-conductors (insulators).
7 Define and draw a graphical illustration of the following:
  (a) direct current;
  (b) alternating current;
  (c) high-frequency current.
8 Explain the following electrical units:
  (a) amps;
  (b) ohms;
  (c) volts;
  (d) watts.
9 Define Ohm's law and use it for calculations.
10 Calculate the cost of electricity by reading the meter for number of units used.
11 Distinguish between closed circuit, open circuit and short circuit.
12 Explain how the following devices modify current:
  (a) transformer;
  (b) rectifier;
  (c) capacitor.
13 Name two types of fuse and give examples of where each may be found.
14 Discuss the replacement of 'blown' fuses.
15 Explain the procedure to be followed when rewiring a plug.

This chapter deals with basic science which is relevant to the beauty therapist. It is suggested that all students study this chapter before embarking on electrical treatments as it will provide a background knowledge of atoms, ions, basic electricity, conductors, electrical units, Ohm's law, devices for modifying current, type of current and circuits. Where relevant, further scientific theory is to be found at the beginning of each chapter.

States of matter

Everything around us is composed of matter and all matter is made up of small particles called atoms. Matter can exist in any one of three states depending on temperature and pressure. The three states of matter are:

1 solid;
2 liquid;
3 gas.

In the solid state, the particles are tightly packed and regularly arranged and move only slightly or vibrate; solids are very dense. In the liquid state, the particles are more widely spaced and move more freely; liquids are usually less dense than solids (ice being one exception). In the gaseous state, the particles are very widely spaced and move at high speed; gases have a lower density than liquids and solids.

Figure 1.2 *Particles in a solid, liquid and a gas*

Solid	Liquid	Gas
		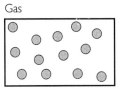
Particles have a regular pattern, are close together, they move slightly and have high density	Particles are more widely spaced, move more freely and have a medium density	Particles are widely spaced, move randomly at high speed and have a low density

If a solid is heated beyond its melting point it will form a liquid, and if a liquid is heated beyond its boiling point it will form a gas. The converse is also true: if a gas is cooled it will condense to form a liquid, and if a liquid is cooled it will form a solid.

Elements

Matter is made up of chemical *elements* and their various compounds. An **element** is a substance in its simplest form which cannot be further broken down by chemical reaction.

There are 109 known elements, and about 90 of these occur naturally. At room temperature and pressure, most elements are solid and metallic, eg copper, iron; some are liquid, eg mercury, bromine; and some are gases, eg hydrogen, oxygen.

Table A *Common elements*

Metal	Non-metal
Copper	Oxygen
Iron	Nitrogen
Zinc	Carbon
Sodium	Chlorine
Potassium	Sulphur
Calcium	

Compounds

Elements can combine and react together to form *compounds*. The properties of the compound will be different from the properties of the individual elements from which it is made, eg the elements hydrogen and oxygen react to form the compound water.

Each element can be represented in shorthand by a symbol usually made up of one or two letters, eg:

Hydrogen, H   Calcium, Ca
Oxygen, O   Chlorine, Cl
Potassium, K   Sodium, Na

When two elements join together to form a compound, the symbols are combined, eg:

Sodium + chlorine → Sodium chloride
$Na^+ + Cl^-$ → NaCl

Atomic structure

Elements are made up of atoms. An atom is the smallest part of an element that retains its distinct chemical properties and that can take part in a chemical reaction. Atoms are made up of even smaller particles, the main ones being protons, electrons and neutrons.

Two of these subatomic particles carry an electrical charge: protons have a positive charge; electrons have a negative charge; neutrons have no charge, ie are neutral.

All the atoms of one element are identical and contain the same numbers of these particles (eg all atoms of helium have two electrons, two protons and two neutrons). Atoms of different elements have different numbers of particles. The arrangement of these particles in an atom follows a definite pattern.

In each atom the protons and neutrons are tightly packed together in the nucleus of the atom. The electrons orbit around the nucleus in distinct energy levels or electron shells. Each orbit or energy level is capable of holding only a certain number of electrons:

- The 1st level holds up to two electrons maximum but can hold less.
- The 2nd level holds up to eight electrons maximum but can hold less.
- The 3rd level holds up to eight electrons maximum but can hold less.
- Further energy levels hold progressively larger numbers.

Because opposite charges attract each other, the negatively charged electrons are held in their orbits by the positive charge of the protons in the nucleus. In every atom the number of positively charged protons is equal to the number of negatively charged

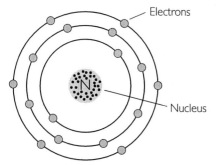

The Nucleus contains 16 protons and 16 neutrons tightly packed together. The 16 electrons move rapidly around the nucleus at distinct energy levels

Figure 1.3   *The arrangement of particles in an atom of oxygen* electrons, therefore the atom has no overall charge; it is electrically neutral.

- 1st level has two therefore is full.
- 2nd level has eight therefore is full.
- 3rd level has six therefore is not full (it could hold 8).

Atoms of different elements combine by chemical reactions to form compounds. Atoms with the maximum number of electrons in their outer shell are said to be stable. They do not readily react with other elements, eg:

Helium (He) has two protons, two neutrons and two electrons. Neon (Ne) has ten protons, ten neutrons and ten electrons.

Figure 1.4   *Stable atoms*

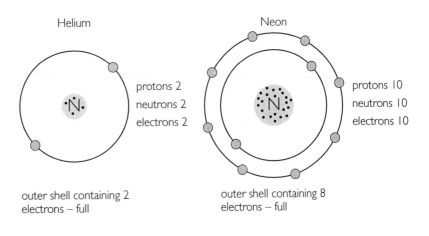

On the other hand, some atoms contain less than the maximum number of electrons in their outer shell and are, therefore, more reactive.

Figure 1.5   *Reactive atoms*

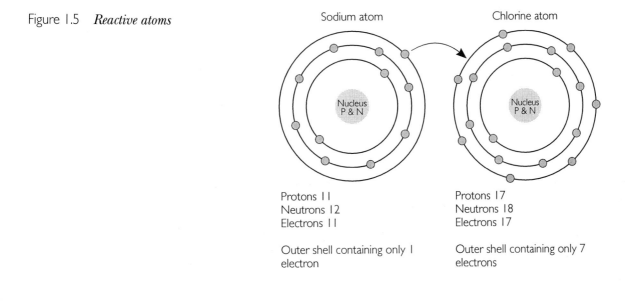

Reactive atoms have a great 'desire' to have the maximum number of electrons in their outer shell. In order to achieve a stable electron pattern, they are able to gain or lose electrons by reacting with other elements to form compounds. The sodium atom has one electron in its outer shell; it needs to lose this to gain a stable electron pattern of eight in the outer shell. The chlorine atom has seven electrons in its outer shell; it needs to gain an electron to give the maximum eight electrons in its outer shell. Sodium and chlorine will therefore readily react together – sodium giving an electron and chlorine receiving an electron. The compound thus formed will be sodium chloride:

$$Na^+ + Cl^- \rightarrow NaCl$$

Ions

Figure 1.6   *Ions*

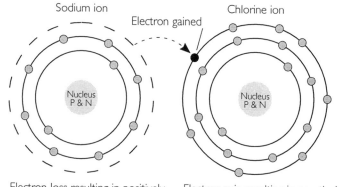

Electron loss resulting in positively charged ion

Electron gain resulting in negatively charged ion

When the sodium atom loses its electron from the outer shell, it will have one more proton than electron, will have a positive charge, and will be called an *ion*. A positively charged ion is called a *cation* (+).

When the chlorine atom gains an electron, it will have one more electron than proton, will have a negative charge, and will be called an ion. A negatively charged *ion* is called an *anion* (−).

This taking and giving of electrons will apply to all reactive atoms and the following principles also apply:

● When an atom gains or loses electrons it becomes a charged particle called an ion.

● If an atom loses electrons it becomes a positively charged ion called a cation.

● If an atom gains electrons it becomes a negatively charged ion called an anion.

(This is easy to remember by taking the first two letters of *an*ion giving *a n*egative *ion*.)

Ions react with each other according to definite laws:

- Ions with the same charge repel.
- Ions with the opposite charge will attract.

(Remember this as it is the fundamental principle on which some galvanic treatments work.)

Electricity

Electricity is the movement of electrons from one atom to another. It may be static or dynamic. Electricity can be produced in three ways:

1 Static electricity produced by friction.
2 Current or dynamic electricity produced by chemical reactions.
3 Current or dynamic electricity produced by magnetic fields.

STATIC ELECTRICITY

Certain substances when rubbed together produce electrical charges or static electricity. The electrons from one material can be transferred to the other material. The material losing electrons becomes positively charged, while the one gaining electrons becomes negatively charged. Remember, these charges obey certain laws of physics: like charges repel each other, while opposite charges attract each other.

This can be demonstrated when brushing hair. The friction of brushing removes electrons from the atoms of the hair. These electrons collect on the brush giving it a negative charge. Loss of electrons leave the hair with a positive charge. Since like charges repel and opposite charges attract, the hairs will fly apart, but will be attracted to the brush. Small crackling noises will be heard and sparks seen in the dark as energy is released.

CURRENT ELECTRICITY

An electric current is a flow of free electrons through a material called a conductor; it flows from an area of excess of electrons to an area of deficiency. In order to achieve current flow a potential difference (PD) or electric force must exist between two ends of the conductor. This force is measured in volts. Some materials, such as metals, are good conductors of electrical charge. This is because the electrons in their outer shell are weakly attached to their atoms and can easily be made to flow through the material.

Figure 1.7   *Electrons flowing through a length of wire*

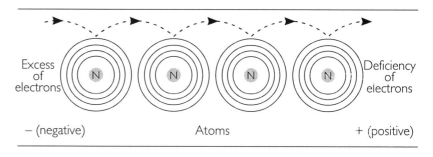

In other materials, the electrons are firmly held to their atoms, are reluctant to be detached and cannot be made to flow through the material. These are non-conductors or insulators. All materials offer some resistance or impedance to the flow of current.

As previously stated, the flow of electrons through the conductor requires a potential difference (PD) to exist between the ends of the wire. This is sometimes called the electromotive force (EMF) and is measured in *volts*. The greater the force, the greater the intensity of the current. This force can be provided by chemical reactions in batteries or cells; or by using magnetic fields in generators.

Table B *Examples of conductors and insulators*

Conductors	Insulators
Copper	Rubber
Zinc	Plastic
Carbon	Glass
Brass	Dry wood

PRODUCTION OF ELECTRICITY BY CHEMICAL REACTION

A simple cell or battery is a means of converting chemical energy into electrical energy. When two different metals called electrodes are immersed in a chemical called an electrolyte, an electric current is produced. The electrolyte is a chemical compound which dissociates into ions when dissolved in water. These ions move towards or away from the electrodes, depending upon their charge.

The metal which is higher in the activity series (in this case the zinc) becomes the negative electrode having an excess of electrons; the other electrode (in this case the carbon) becomes the positive electrode having a deficiency of electrons. Therefore electrons will flow through the wire from the zinc electrode to the carbon electrode. This flow of electrons will continue until all the chemicals in the electrolyte are used up, at which time the current flow will stop.

Figure 1.8   *A simple cell*

Dry cell batteries, being easily transportable, are now widely used to power radios, torches and portable beauty therapy equipment.

Figure 1.9 *Structure of a dry battery*

The principle of how they work is the same as described above, but their construction is different. The electrolyte is a paste contained within a zinc electrode casing; the carbon rod electrode is placed down the centre. As the chemicals are used up, the battery becomes 'flat' and is disposed of.

Rechargeable batteries are available, which may be recharged by connecting them to a mains-powered battery charger. They are usually left on overnight to recharge and can then be re-used when required.

The type of current produced by cells and batteries always flows in the same direction and is called direct current (DC) or constant current.

Figure 1.10 *Direct current flowing in one direction*

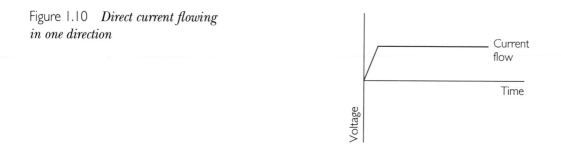

ELECTRICITY BY ELECTRO-MAGNETIC INDUCTION

Electricity obtained from the mains is produced by a dynamo or generator in large power stations. It is produced using magnetism. When a coil of wire is rotated between the north and south poles of a magnet, it cuts through the magnetic lines of force or the magnetic field, an electromagnetic force (EMF) is produced in the coil, ie electrons will flow through the wire. An EMF can also be induced by moving a magnet through a coil of wire.

Figure 1.11 *Rotating coil cutting through the lines of force*

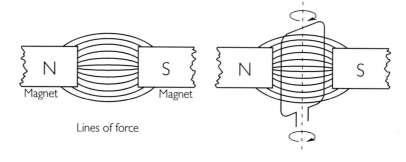

Rotating coil will cut through the lines of force

Each power station will have a number of these generators for producing electricity. The long coils of wire are rotated by water power or by steam from boilers heated by coal, oil or nuclear energy. Each coil of wire is rotated at speed between the poles of a large magnet.

As the coil rotates, it cuts through the lines of force each half revolution, and this produces an alternating current. Beginning at zero, the current rises to a maximum positive value, falls to zero and then rises to a maximum negative value and returns to zero with each revolution.

Figure 1.12   *Alternating current reversing each half cycle*

One complete revolution is known as a cycle. Half the cycle will rise to maximum positive and half to maximum negative. The number of these cycles produced per second is known as the frequency of the current. The unit of frequency is the *hertz* (Hz).

The frequency of the mains supply in the United Kingdom (UK) is 50 Hz (ie 50 cycles of current flow every second when current is switched on at the mains). A current can be made to oscillate at very high frequencies when the cycles are very close together.

Figure 1.13   *Alternating current of higher frequency*

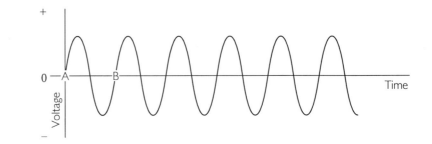

The voltage produced at power stations is high at 11,000 volts. It is further increased and then reduced for mains supply to 240 volts. The mains voltage is different on the Continent.

Electrical units

As explained above, the pressure or force required to drive a current around a circuit is known as the potential difference (PD) or electromotive force, and is measured in volts often referred to as voltage (a voltmeter is used to measure voltage).

The intensity of the current or rate of flow of the current is measured in *amps* or amperes (an ammeter is used to measure amperage.)

Any conductor offers resistance to a current passing along it, this resistance is measured in *ohms*. (The longer the length of conductor, the greater the resistance. The thinner the conductor the greater the resistance.)

The intensity of the current

The intensity of a current is the number of electrons (amps) passing one point in one second. It depends on two factors:

1 The potential difference, ie the amount of force (volts).
2 The resistance offered to the current (ohms).

The relationship between current flow (amps), potential difference (volts) and resistance (ohms) is expressed by Ohm's law.

Ohm's law

This states that the current flowing through a circuit varies in direct proportion to the potential difference and in inverse proportion to the resistance.

ie current (amps) $= \dfrac{\text{potential difference (volts)}}{\text{resistance (ohms)}}$

or
$$I = \frac{V}{R}$$

This means that if the PD increases, the current increases, but if the resistance increases, the current decreases. Using this formula, it is possible to calculate any one unit providing the other two are known.

Example: if the voltage is 200 volts and the resistance is 40 ohms, calculate the current.

I   is the current in amps.
V   is the potential difference or voltage measured in volts.
R   is the resistance measured in ohms.

$$I = \frac{V}{R}$$

$$I = \frac{200}{40}$$

I = 50 amps

Or, if the resistance is 40 ohms and the current is 50 amps, calculate the voltage.

V = I × R
V = 50 × 40
V = 200 volts

Or, if the current is 50 amps and the voltage is 200 volts, calculate the resistance.

$$R = \frac{V}{I}$$

$$R = \frac{200}{50}$$

R = 40 ohms

It is easier to remember the formula by drawing a triangle:

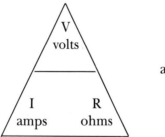

$$amps = \frac{volts}{ohms}$$

volts = amps × ohms

$$ohms = \frac{volts}{amps}$$

Cover one unit and the other side of the equation is given by the position of the other two units.

Power

The power used when running electrical equipment is measured in watts.

> power = current × voltage

or

> watts = amps × volts

Example: the power supplied by a socket, 15 amps × 240 volts will be:

> watts = 15 × 240 = 3,600 watts (1,000 watts is 1 kilowatt)

Cost of electricity

The power of an appliance and the time for which it is used determines the amount of electricity used by that appliance. This quantity is measured in kilowatt-hours (kWh). (A kW appliance running for 1 hour uses 1 kilowatt-hour.)

The Electricity Board charges a fixed amount for each kilowatt-hour, which are known as units of electricity used. The number of units used by a house or salon are registered on an electric meter which forms part of the mains circuit. Older meters consist of four dials which register thousands, hundreds, tens and units, but the more modern meters have a digital display showing the number of units used.

Figure 1.14   *Electricity meter with dials*

The reading indicated above is 2150 units.

The cost of electricity is calculated by reading the meter and multiplying the number of units used by the cost per unit:

Cost of electricity = number of units × cost per unit
                      (number of kilowatt hours)

Circuits

The pathway taken by an electric current is known as a *circuit*. In order for the current to flow, this pathway must be complete from one terminal of the electrical source to the other. If it is broken, the current flow will stop.

A closed circuit is an unbroken pathway between the negative and positive terminals of an electrical source. The current flows continuously in a closed circuit.

An open circuit is a pathway which is broken or interrupted by a switch or other device. This breaks the connection and stops the flow of current.

A short circuit occurs when the current does not pass around its designated course but takes a short cut through a path of least resistance, eg across a break in insulation.

Components or devices used in circuits to modify (change) currents

It is necessary to modify currents used in beauty therapy equipment. Batteries do not supply direct current (DC) at a high enough voltage for all treatment purposes, therefore mains current (AC) is used and modified.

TRANSFORMER

A transformer is a device for altering the voltage in alternating current circuits. The voltage may be increased using a step up transformer *or* the voltage may be decreased using a step down transformer.

A transformer is made of a soft iron core and two coils of wire. The current flows in through the primary coil and out via the secondary coil. If there are a greater number of coils in the secondary wire, the voltage will be stepped up. If there are fewer coils, the voltage will be stepped down.

Figure 1.15 *Step up and step down transformers*

(Remember 'TV': *Transformer changes Voltage*.)

RECTIFIER

A rectifier is a device for changing alternating current to direct current. This process is called rectification. There are two types of rectifier:

1 A half wave rectifier: this blocks impulses in one direction.

Figure 1.16   *Half wave rectifier*

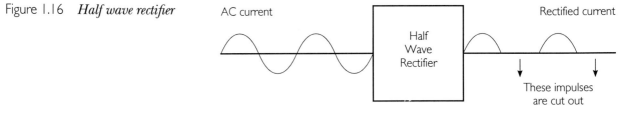

2 A full wave rectifier: this blocks but redirects impulses in one direction.

Figure 1.17   *Full wave rectifier*

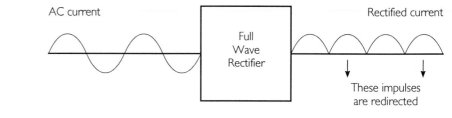

(Remember 'RAC': *R*ectifier changes *A*lternating *C*urrent.)

CAPACITOR OR CONDENSER

A capacitor is a device which stores electrical charge and discharges it when required. It is used to smooth the impulse pattern after rectification.

Figure 1.18   *A capacitor or condenser*

RHEOSTAT OR VARIABLE RESISTANCE

A rheostat is a device used to control the amount of current flowing through a circuit. It varies the resistance; the higher the resistance the weaker the current. It is made of a coil of resistance wire with a sliding contact. It is wired in series with the apparatus.

Figure 1.19   *A rheostat*

If all the resistance wire is included in the circuit (contact at point B), the current will be at its lowest. The current can be increased by moving the contact towards point A. Used in wax pots to control the temperature for melting the wax and in lamps to control the intensity of light.

POTENTIOMETER

A potentiometer is a device for varying the voltage in a circuit. It must be wired in parallel to the circuit, and is used in constant current galvanic machines to control the current during galvanic treatments.

STARTER OR SWITCH

A starter is a device for switching on a current, ie starting the flow of electrons. When the client is correctly attached to the apparatus, closing the switch completes the circuit and the current will flow; when the switch is open, the circuit is broken and the current stops.

Electricity supply

Figure 1.20   *A power station*

Electricity is generated in large power stations at 11,000 volts. It is more efficient to transmit electricity at even higher voltages, and transformers are used to step up the voltage to 400,000 volts. This is transmitted to substations by high-voltage cables suspended on pylons. At the substations more transformers are used to step down the voltage to suit the requirements of factories, etc, and to supply private homes and salons with a voltage of 240 volts.

Mains circuit

Figure 1.21   *Ring–main circuit*

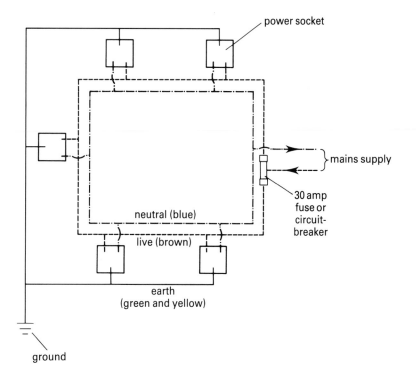

Electricity is supplied to the home via a cable that contains two wires – one live and one neutral – which is earthed at the substation. The mains cable enters the house and passes to a sealed box where the live wire is connected to a fuse. This box can only be opened by engineers from the Electricity Board who must investigate any faults if the fuse should 'blow'.

The mains cable then enters the meter, which registers all the units of electricity used over a period of time. It then enters the fuse box called the consumer unit. This box contains the master switch, fuses and circuit breakers for the ring circuit, lighting circuit and others, such as the immersion heater or cooker. If a fault develops within a circuit, the connected fuse will blow and the current flow will stop. This prevents the wire from overheating and causing fires.

Each appliance is connected to the mains circuit sockets by a flex and a plug. This plug also contains a fuse, which is designed to 'blow' if there is electrical overload or if an appliance develops an electrical fault. When this fuse breaks the circuit, the appliance is effectively disconnected from the mains, but other appliances are not affected.

Fuses

A fuse is a safety device to stop the flow of electricity. It is the weakest point in a circuit. Fuses are found in the consumer unit (fuse box) and in the plugs which connect an appliance to the mains. If a circuit is overloaded, or if the wiring or the appliance are faulty, the fuse will 'blow' – the wire melts, will break the circuit and the flow of electricity will stop. There are two types of fuse:

REWIRABLE FUSES

These are made of short lengths of tinned copper wire held by screws in a porcelain container. They are found in older fuse boxes. Each fuse holder is colour coded with a spot to indicate the current rating of the wire.

CARTRIDGE FUSES

Figure 1.22   *Structure of a cartridge fuse*

These are made of short lengths of tinned copper embedded in sand and contained in a small porcelain or glass tube. The wire is attached to metal caps at each end of the tube. In the fuse box the cartridge is housed in a metal or plastic holder. In the same way as rewirable fuses, these are colour coded to indicate the current rating. It is impossible to fit the wrong cartridge into a holder as each rating is different in size – the higher the rating the larger the cartridge.

Table C *Current ratings for various circuits*

Circuit	Current rating	Colour coding
Lighting	5A	white
Immersion heater	15A	blue
Storage heaters	20A	yellow
Ring main	30A	red
Instant hot water heater	45A	green

To replace a blown fuse, first switch off the mains switch in the fuse box (this must be done to stop the flow of electricity to the premises and make sure that there is no chance of the operator receiving an electric shock which can prove fatal). Disconnect all appliances and check each holder in the fuse box to locate the blown fuse. Then check the relevant appliance to find the cause of the fuse blowing. It may be a fault in the appliance, such as a loose connection, a break in insulation or old, corroded fuse wire. If it is a rewirable fuse, remove the old wire and replace it with a new wire of the same current rating. If it is a cartridge fuse, remove and discard the old fuse and replace it with a new cartridge of the same size and current rating. If a fuse continues to blow, call in an electrician to check the circuit.

PLUG FUSES

These are cartridge-type fuses that are fitted on to the live wire in the plug and are designed to protect the appliance. Plug cartridge fuses are all the same size but they have three different current ratings.

- 3A rating for use with appliances up to 700 watts.
- 5A rating for use with appliances between 700 and 1000 watts.
- 13A rating for use with appliances between 1000 and 3000 watts.

To replace a plug fuse, disconnect the plug from the socket. Open the plug by undoing the main screw. Remove the old cartridge and replace it with a cartridge of the same rating.

Circuit breakers

These are modern devices designed to break the circuit if a fault is present. They may be trip switches or buttons that are designed to switch to the 'off' or 'open' position if the circuit is overloaded or faulty. The circuit breaker can easily be reset after the fault has been found and repaired. This is done by pushing in the button or moving the switch.

Wiring a plug

Figure 1.23   *Wiring of a plug*

Earth terminal
Earth conductor wire
Neutral conductor wire
Neutral terminal
Live terminal
Live conductor wire
Fuse
Outer sheath of supply cord
Cross-bar cord grip

Unscrew and remove the cover, and then examine the plug. There are three connector terminals connecting with each pin that are labelled:

E for earth

L for live

N for neutral

Across the live terminal is the fuse and at the base of the plug is a cord grip. Next examine the flex: this is insulated with a thick outer layer of rubber or plastic; inside are three wires with coloured insulating covers. New flexes have different colour coding from old flexes. The wires should be connected as follows:

Table D   *How the wires should be connected*

Terminal	Colour	Old colour coding
E (earth)	green yellow	green
L (live)	brown	red
N (neutral)	blue	black

Cut back the outer insulation to expose around 4 cm of the inner wires, and then cut the insulation around each wire exposing just over 1 cm of wire at the end – twist the bare wire around. Push the flex under the cord grip and screw the grip down (make sure that the grip holds the insulation) and bend each wire towards the correct terminal. The terminal may have a hole and a screw clamp or may require the wire to be placed around a post and then screwed down. Bend the end of the wire and push it into the hole or twist it in a clockwise direction around the post, and then screw tightly. Make sure that the wires are just the right length to reach their terminals without strain. The insulation should reach the screw. Check that the correct colour wires have been connected to the appropriate terminals. It is most important to connect the earth wire securely as this is a safety device. Should the casing become 'live', the earth wire conducts the current safely to earth, thus preventing a shock if the appliance is touched.

Replace the fuse checking that it is the correct size. Screw the cord grip tightly, replace the cover and screw down tightly.

If an appliance has only two wires, a live and neutral, which are connected to the appropriate L and N terminals, it is still safe to use because manufacturers have ensured that the appliance is double insulated so that no electricity can pass to the user even if there is a fault. These appliances will show the symbol ▭ indicating that it is double insulated.

Sockets

In order to provide the appliance with electricity, the plug must be pushed firmly into the socket and switched on. The socket has three rectangular holes and a switch; the live and neutral holes have shutters. The earth pin on the plug is longer than the other pins – as this is pushed in the shutters move and the other pins can be pushed home. This is a safety device to prevent young children putting fingers or other articles into the live and neutral holes and receiving shocks which could prove to be fatal.

Electrolysis

This involves the passage of direct current through a solution which results in the production of certain chemical reactions. Some chemical compounds dissolve in water to form a solution. When the compounds dissolve, they dissociate (ie split) into ions; either cations (−) or anions (+). These ions increase the conductivity of the solution enabling an electric current to flow easily (a solution that conducts a current is called an electrolyte). If direct current is made to flow through such a solution, the ions will move towards the electrode with the opposite charge.

- The negatively charged electrode is called the *cathode.*
- The positively charged electrode is called the *anode.*

Figure 1.24 *Electrolysis of sodium chloride solution*

When the current is switched on, opposite charges will attract, therefore:

- The cations (+) will move towards the cathode (−). This is known as *cataphoresis*.
- The anions (−) will move towards the anode (+). This is known as *anaphoresis*.

The chemical reactions at these electrodes will depend upon the chemical composition of the electrolyte and the electrodes.

Currents used in beauty therapy

GALVANIC CURRENT

A direct current is used in galvanic treatments and also for epilation. The direct current flows in one direction only and has polarity. When the current is flowing, one electrode will always be negatively charged (the cathode); the other will be positively charged (the anode). The treatments using direct current are shown in Table E.

Table E *Treatments using direct current*

Facial work	*Body work*
Disincrustation	Body galvanism
Iontophoresis (see page 98)	Iontophoresis

HIGH-FREQUENCY TREATMENTS

These use a high-frequency alternating current of around 250,000 Hz to improve the condition of the skin. There are two methods of application:

- The direct method
- The indirect method or Viennese massage (see page 29).

MUSCLE STIMULATING CURRENTS

These are variable currents of sufficient intensity and duration to stimulate motor nerves and produce contraction of muscles. The current may be modified low-frequency alternating current or more usually, modified direct current. A variety of pulses can be produced – these are arranged in 'trains' with rest periods in between. When the current flows, the muscle contracts; when the current stops, the muscle relaxes – this stimulates normal movement.

INTERFERENTIAL CURRENT

Two high-frequency alternating currents are applied diagonally to the same area of tissue. The effect on the tissue is produced by an interferential current whose frequency is the difference between the frequencies of the current applied.

Electricity in beauty therapy

The beauty therapist uses a variety of equipment powered by electricity:

1 Vacuum suction machines: electrical energy is used to drive a motor which produces reduced pressure within glass or plastic cups that are applied to the body.
2 Mechanical massage: electrical energy is used to drive a motor which, via a shank, moves various heads. Equipment used for mechanical massage includes:
   (a) Gyratory vibrators – both hand-held and floor models.
   (b) Percussion vibrator with its up-and-down tapping movement.
   (c) Belt massager where vibratory movements are produced along the belt.

(d) Audio-sonic vibrator where a coil is made to vibrate to and fro, this is transferred through an applicator head on to the tissues. The frequency of the vibrations is within the audible range and a low humming sound can be heard when in use.

3 Heat lamps: when an electric current flows through a wire of high resistance, heat is produced. This heating effect is used in both luminous and non-luminous heat lamps.

4 Steam treatments: facial steamers and steam baths. A heating element is used to heat water in a container to produce steam.

5 Wax treatments: heating elements are used to melt wax and bring it to the required temperature of 49°C.

6 Ultraviolet lamps and sunbeds: an electric current is used to power mercury vapour lamps and sunbed tubes to produce ultraviolet light. It is used mainly for its tanning effects, but can be used to treat acne, psoriasis, wounds, etc.

Safety considerations when using electrical equipment

1 Always buy equipment from a reputable dealer, who can provide a good, reliable backup service.

2 Ensure that all equipment is regularly maintained and in good working order.

3 Ensure that insulation is sound, with no breaks or worn patches.

4 Ensure that all connections, such as leads, terminals and plugs, are sound and secure.

5 Replace fuses when necessary with those of the correct rating. If a fuse blows repeatedly, do not replace it with one of a higher rating, but seek advice from electrician.

6 Do not overload the circuit by using multi-blocks, etc.

7 Keep electrical equipment away from water. Take particular care if pads have to be moistened with water, and do not allow water to drip over the machine.

8 Do not touch electrical equipment or leads, plugs, etc, with wet hands.

9 Make sure the equipment is stable and not in a position where it may easily be pushed or topple over.

10 Ensure that flexes do not trail over the working area.

11 Always test the current on yourself before applying it to the client.

12 Cover equipment when not in use to keep free from dust.

13 Remove any faulty equipment from the working area and label it clearly with: **Faulty – do not use**.

SUMMARY

STATES OF MATTER

- The three states of matter are: solid, liquid and gas.
- All matter can exist in any one of these states, depending upon temperature and pressure.

ELEMENTS

- Matter is made up of chemical elements.
- An element is a substance in its simplest form – it cannot be further broken down by chemical reaction.
- There are 109 known elements.
- Examples include oxygen, carbon, copper, iron.

COMPOUNDS

- A compound is formed when elements react and combine together to form a new substance.

ATOMS

- An atom is the smallest part of an element which retains its distinct chemical properties and which can take part in a chemical reaction.
- An atom has a nucleus containing protons with a positive charge, and neutrons with no charge. Electrons with a negative charge orbit around the nucleus at different energy levels.

DEFINITIONS

- Protons are positively charged particles found in the nucleus of an atom.
- Neutrons are neutral particles (ie have no charge) found in the nucleus of an atom.
- Electrons are negatively charged particles found orbiting the nucleus at different energy levels. There are up to two electrons in the first level, and up to eight in the second and third levels, etc.
- All the atoms of an element are identical, having the same number of neutrons, protons and electrons.

- Elements are different from each other because of the different numbers of particles in their atoms.

IONS

- When atoms gain or lose electrons from their outer shell or energy level, they become ions.
- If an atom loses electrons, it becomes a positively charged ion called a *cation.*
- If an atom gains electrons, it becomes a negatively charged ion called an *anion.*

ELECTRICITY

- Electricity is the movement of electrons from one atom to another. It may be static electricity, or it may be made to move through a conductor (known as dynamic or current electricity).
- When rubbed together, substances produce static electricity.
- Dynamic electricity is produced chemically by cells and batteries, or it may be produced by magnetic fields in generators.

CURRENT ELECTRICITY

- An electric current is a flow of free electrons through a material called a conductor, from an area where electrons are in excess to an area deficient in electrons.
- The amount of current flowing is measured in *amps.*

POTENTIAL DIFFERENCE (PD) OR ELECTROMOTIVE FORCE

- This is the force required to achieve a flow of electricity through a conductor.
- Known as voltage, it is measured in volts.

RESISTANCE

- All conductors have a tendency to resist the flow of electrons.
- Electrical resistance is measured in ohms.
- The relationship between current flow (amps), potential difference (volts) and resistance (ohms) is expressed by Ohm's law.

Ohm's law

- This states that the current flowing through a circuit varies in direct proportion to the potential difference and in inverse proportion to the resistance.

$$I = \frac{V}{R}$$

Power

- The unit of power is the watt:

  watts = amps × volts

Direct current

- Cells and batteries produce direct current (DC).
- Direct current flows in one direction only, without variation. It has polarity.
- One electrode will be negatively charged (the cathode) and the other will be positively charged (the anode).

Alternating current

- Generators produce alternating current (AC).
- Beginning at zero, the current rises to maximum positive value, falls to zero and then rises to maximum negative value and returns to zero. This is one cycle.
- The number of cycles per second is the frequency and is measured in hertz (Hz).
- The frequency of the UK mains is 50 Hz.
- Alternating current from the mains can be modified to provide the direct current necessary for some treatments.

Devices for modifying current

- A transformer changes voltage in AC circuits.
- It may be a step up transformer for increasing voltage, or a step down transformer for decreasing voltage.
- A rectifier changes AC to DC, it may be a half wave rectifier or full wave rectifier.

- A capacitor or condenser stores electrical charge and discharges it when required.
- A rheostat or variable resistance varies the current flowing in a circuit. It varies the resistance – the higher the resistance the weaker the current.
- A potentiometer varies the voltage in the circuit.

FUSES

- A fuse is designed to be the weakest point in the circuit.
- It is a safety device to stop the flow of current should the circuit or appliance be faulty.
- There are two types: rewirable fuse and cartridge fuse.

COLOUR CODING OF PLUGS

- (see page 20)

QUESTIONS

1 Explain the difference between the following: solids, liquids and gases.
2 Define the term 'element' and give two examples.
3 Draw a diagram showing the structure of an atom. Label and give the electrical charge of each particle.
4 Define the following terms:
  (a) ion,
  (b) cation,
  (c) anion.
5 Complete the following statements:
  (a) Ions with the same charge . . .
  (b) Ions with the opposite charge . . .
6 Give two ways in which dynamic electricity is produced.
7 Explain how electricity flows through a conductor.
8 Which of the following are good conductors of electricity:
  (a) copper,
  (b) carbon,
  (c) plastic,
  (d) brass,
  (e) glass,
  (f) dry wood.
9 Explain the difference between DC and AC. Draw a simple diagram to illustrate each one.
10 Explain the meaning of the following:
  (a) high frequency current,
  (b) polarity,
  (c) electrodes,
  (d) electrolyte.
11 State Ohm's law.
12 If the resistance in a circuit increases, what happens to the current flow?
13 If the resistance in a circuit is 30 ohms and the voltage is 240 volts, calculate the current flowing around the circuit.
14 Explain the function of the following devices in a circuit:
  (a) transformer,
  (b) rectifier.
15 Explain the purpose of a fuse.
16 Name the types of fuses available and indicate where they may be found.
17 List the terminals found in a plug and indicate the new colour coding of connecting wires.

CHAPTER 2

High frequency treatment

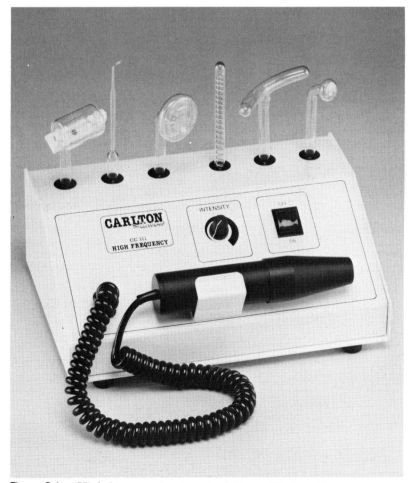

Figure 2.1   *High frequency treatment machine with electrodes*

OBJECTIVES

After you have studied this chapter you will be able to:

1 Identify the terminals on the machine.
2 Identify the electrodes used for each method of application.
3 Differentiate between the effects of the direct and indirect methods of application.
4 Select the appropriate method of application to meet the needs of the client.
5 Identify the contra-indications to treatment.
6 Treat the client paying due consideration to maximum efficiency, comfort, safety and hygiene.

Figure 2.1 is a photograph of a high frequency treatment machine and the electrodes used to deliver the current to the client. As its name implies, this machine uses a high frequency current (a current which alternates at over 100,000 cycles per second is known as high frequency). The high frequency output of these machines is an alternating current of around 250,000 Hz at a high voltage but low current flow. This alternating current will not stimulate muscle contraction because the duration of the pulses is too short. It passes easily through the skin to produce heating effects.

There are two methods of application:

1 the direct method, and
2 the indirect method (Viennese massage).

These two methods have different effects on the tissues and must be selected carefully to suit the client. They are primarily used on the face but may also be used on the body – the technique, effects, etc, are similar for both.

Machines

Machines producing high frequency currents require only two controls: an on/off switch and an intensity control. The current is delivered to the client by means of one electrode; different electrodes are used for the direct and indirect methods of application.

Electrodes used in treatment

Figure 2.2   *Electrodes used for direct high frequency treatment*

ELECTRODES USED FOR THE DIRECT METHOD

Shown above is a variety of electrodes shaped for specific purposes. They are made of glass with metal end connections. A very small amount of air, neon or mercury, is sealed inside the tube. When the electrode is pushed into its holder, the metal end makes contact with a metal plate in the holder. When the current is switched on, it flows from the machine, through the holder, to the electrode. The air or gas inside the tube ionises, the current flows through the tube and is dispersed into the tissues under the electrode. The electrodes glow violet if they contain air or orange if they contain neon. If they contain mercury vapour, they will glow a blue-violet colour and give off ultraviolet rays. Most of these rays will not pass through the tubes as they are made of glass, which absorbs ultraviolet radiation. A metal electrode is sometimes found inside the glass which intensifies the effect.

THE ELECTRODE USED FOR THE INDIRECT METHOD

Saturator held in the hand   Holder held in other hand

Figure 2.3   *Electrode used for indirect high frequency treatment*

This is known as a saturator. It may be made of metal or glass and again fits into a holder. The client holds the holder in one hand and the saturator is held firmly in the other hand.

The current passes through the holder into the saturator and 'charges' the client. The therapist massages the client and the current is 'drawn off' through the therapist's fingers. The therapist is part of the circuit when giving this treatment.

Note: Rings must not be worn on the hand that holds the saturator.

The direct method

This method is particularly suitable for the client with greasy, seborrhoeic, acne prone skin due to its stimulating, drying effect. It may also be used on dry and mature skin. (The treatment time for this type of skin must be short – around 5 minutes – otherwise the condition will be exacerbated.)

This method uses a glass electrode which is moved slowly over the skin; it is sometimes known as *effluvation*. The current passes from the electrode and is dispersed over the skin. The warmth generated in the tissues will produce the beneficial effects for the client. The sparking is used for its germicidal effect.

Figures 2.4 and 2.5   *Treatment using direct high frequency. The glass electrode is moved slowly all over the face and neck with rhythmical, circular movements. Contact with the skin must be maintained throughout. The more superficial the movement, the greater the stimulation. Place the other hand on the bed or hold the cable.*

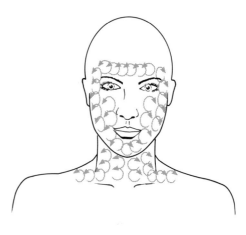

Uses

1 To dry and improve the condition of seborrhoeic skin.
2 To dry greasy skins and greasy areas on a combination skin (dry/greasy skin).
3 To improve the condition of blemished skin.
4 To destroy bacteria and aid healing of acne and pustular prone skin by means of sparking.
5 To increase sebaceous secretions on a dry, mature skin. In order to achieve this, the treatment is carried out for a short time only (4–5 minutes) and uses the warmth created by the current (too long a treatment will increase the dryness).

Effects

1 *Production of heat.* The rapidly oscillating current produces rapid motion of the molecules in the tissues which generates heat.

This heating is greatest in the superficial tissues under the electrode.

2 *Increased metabolic rate.* Metabolism is a chemical reaction capable of being accelerated by heat. An increase in metabolic rate creates a demand for oxygen and nutrients and an increase in output of waste products. This promotes healing and improves the condition of the skin.

3 *Vasodilation resulting in hyperaemia and erythema.* Heat causes vasodilation and an increase in the flow of blood to the area. The increase in metabolism produces an increase in metabolites which act on capillary walls producing dilation; this also increases the blood supply. In this way, oxygen and nutrients are brought more rapidly to the area and waste products are carried away. This improves the condition of the skin.

4 *Soothing effects on nerves.* Mild heat has a soothing effect on nerve endings, producing a feeling of relaxtion.

5 *Increased activity of sebaceous glands.* Warmth increases the activity of sebaceous glands. This aids the release of blockages caused by build up of sebum. It increases the lubrication of dry, dehydrated skins.

6 *Germicidal effect.* When the electrode is held just off the skin (no more than 7 mm or $\frac{1}{4}$ in away) the current jumps across the gap forming a spark. The oxygen in the air is ionised and forms ozone, which destroys bacteria and promotes the healing of papules and pustules. As the current jumps, the spark produces ultraviolet rays, which destroy bacteria. The sparking itself may burn and destroy bacteria. Great care must be taken when sparking as too large a gap and too long a spark can destroy the tissues. This effect can be used medically for the removal of warts, skin tags, etc. It is known as *fulguration.*

7 *Drying effects.* The sparks stimulate nerve endings in the skin, which result in the constricting of the pores. Oxygen in the air is converted to ozone, which has the drying effect.

Contra-indications

1 Cuts and abrasions.
2 Vascular conditions.
3 Hairy areas.
4 Metal fillings (excessive) or heavy bridge work.
5 Sinus blockages.
6 Tense, nervous clients upset by the noise of the machine.
7 Skin disorders/diseases.

DANGERS

1 The main danger with high frequency current is shock. Shock may be caused in the following ways:
   (a) Touching faulty apparatus.
   (b) Wearing jewellery during treatment.
   (c) Touching metal objects which earths the current.
   (d) Lifting the electrode off the skin during treatment.
   (e) Placing the electrode on the skin after the intensity is turned up and lifting it off the skin before the intensity is turned down.
2 Destruction of tissues if sparking is at too great a distance and for too long a time.

PRECAUTIONS

1 Remove all metal and jewellery from the treatment area.
2 Ensure that the client is not touching any metal, such as the frame of the couch.
3 Warn the client of the machine's noise and explain the treatment.
4 Always keep the electrode in contact with the client.
5 Do not use skin lotions containing alcohol as alcohol is highly flammable (although the danger of igniting it is extremely small).
6 Do not spark more than 7 mm ($\frac{1}{4}$ in) away from the skin surface as this is destructive to tissues.
7 Speak to the client during the treatment.

TREATMENT TECHNIQUE

PREPARATION OF THE CLIENT

1 Place the client in a well-supported and comfortable position.
2 Check that all jewellery has been removed.
3 Check for contra-indications.
4 Explain the treatment to the client, tell her of the noise produced by the machine and reassure her as necessary.
5 Cleanse the skin but do not use a toner containing alcohol.
6 Apply talc or ozone cream to the face and neck to facilitate movement of electrode, or apply a clean gauze rectangle.

PROCEDURE

1 Place the machine on suitable, stable base and check the plugs and leads.
2 Check the intensity control is at zero.

3 Collect all commodities.

4 Test the machine.

5 Select a suitable electrode and clean it with a disinfectant wipe.

6 Place the electrode on the client's face, switch on the machine and increase the intensity up to the client's tolerance. This may have to be decreased over bony areas.

7 Massage in broad circular movements over the face and neck without breaking contact with the skin. The more superficial the movement, the greater the stimulation.

8 Spark if necessary (the electrode may need changing).

9 Lower the intensity to zero and switch off the machine before removing the electrode from the client's face.

10 Remove the medium and tone the skin.

11 Clean the electrode carefully by wiping with hot water and detergent and then a disinfectant wipe. Take particular care not to wet the metal contact.

TIMING OF TREATMENTS

- Oily skin: 10–15 minutes
- Dry, dehydrated skin: 3–5 minutes

The indirect method or Viennese massage

This method is used for clients with dry, lined and dehydrated skin. This method uses a saturator which is held firmly in the client's hand. The holder is held in the other hand (see Figure 2.3). When the current is switched on, it flows through the saturator and charges the client; the therapist massages the client's face and the current discharges from the face to the massaging fingers. The therapist is part of the circuit during indirect high frequency treatments. This is a warming and relaxing treatment.

Figures 2.6 and 2.7 *Treatment with indirect high frequency. The hands are moved slowly over the face and neck with rhythmical, circular movements. One hand must always remain in contact with the face. The more superficial the movement, the greater the stimulation.*

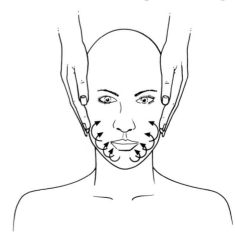

USES

1 To improve the condition of dry, dehydrated skin.
2 To improve sluggish circulation.
3 To improve the condition of tired skin with fine lines.
4 To promote the relaxation of tissues.

EFFECTS

1 Warmth is produced in the superficial tissues.
2 Vasodilation of surface capillaries producing hyperaemia and erythema.
3 The increase in blood flow to the area will bring nutrients and oxygen to nourish the tissues and will remove waste products. This will improve the condition of tissues.
4 The increase in metabolic rate due to heating will also improve the condition of the skin.
5 The mild warmth and slow massage has a sedative effect on the sensory nerve endings and produces relaxation of the tissues.
6 The friction produced by the massage movements aids desquamation (loss of dead skin).

CONTRA-INDICATIONS

1 Hypersensitive skin.
2 Vascular conditions.
3 Cuts and abrasions.
4 Skin diseases/disorders.

DANGERS

Shock as for direct high frequency treatment.

PRECAUTIONS

1 Remove all jewellery and metal. If the client is unable or unwilling to remove a wedding ring, the holder can be held in the ringed hand and the saturator in the hand free of jewellery.
2 Ensure that the client is not touching any metal.
3 Warn the client of the noise from the machine.
4 The client must be told to hold the saturator firmly – one hand holding the holder and the other holding the saturator firmly (sparks will occur if the saturator is loosely held.)
5 Put talc on the hand.
6 Always keep one hand in contact with the client when turning the machine on and off. Remember that removing one hand

from the face intensifies the current through the other hand, and avoid creating discomfort especially over bony areas, such as the forehead.

7 Speak to the client during the treatment.

TREATMENT TECHNIQUE

PREPARATION OF THE CLIENT

1 Place the client in a well-supported and comfortable position.
2 Check that all jewellery has been removed.
3 Check for contra-indications.
4 Explain the treatment to the client, tell her of the noise produced by the machine and reassure her as necessary.
5 Cleanse the skin.
6 Apply talc to the face and neck for a superficial and more stimulating effect. Apply cream for a soothing, relaxing effect.

PROCEDURE

1 Place the machine on a suitable stable base and check all plugs and leads.
2 Check that the intensity controls are at zero.
3 Collect all commodities.
4 Test the machine.
5 Wipe the saturator with a disinfectant wipe and ask the client to hold the saturator firmly. If necessary, talc the hand to absorb any perspiration.
6 Place one hand on the client's face and, using small circular movements, begin to massage the area.
7 Turn the machine up slowly within the client's tolerance.
8 Place the other hand on the opposite side of the face and massage slowly with both hands. Warmth should be felt in the fingers.
9 Do not lose contact with both hands as this will result in a shock to the client.
10 At the end of the treatment, remove one hand from the client's face, reduce the current intensity slowly to zero and switch off the machine.
11 Remove the cream or talc.
12 Clean the saturator carefully by wiping with hot water and detergent and then with a disinfectant wipe. Take particular care not to wet the metal contact.

Figure 2.8 *High frequency unit with electrodes*

TIMING OF TREATMENT

Eight–20 minutes depending on client's skin type and tolerance.

SUMMARY

- A high frequency current is a rapidly oscillating current of over 100,000 Hz (cycles per second).
- The frequency produced by beauty therapy equipment is around 250,000 Hz.
- It passes easily through the skin to produce heating effects.
- It will not stimulate muscles to contract as the frequency is too high and, therefore, the pulse duration is too short.
- High frequency current may be applied to the body in two ways: the direct method and the indirect method (Viennese massage).

THE DIRECT METHOD

- With the direct method, the current is applied to the skin by means of a glass electrode. It is used for its warming and stimulating effects. Sparking is used for its germicidal effect. Sparking must be carried out with care, it must be done quickly and the gap between the electrode and the skin should be less than 7 mm or $\frac{1}{4}$ in. If sparking is done slowly and with too big a gap, the tissues may be destroyed.
- Skin types that benefit from direct high frequency treatment are: greasy seborrhoeic skin; blemished skin with papules and pustules; a sluggish skin; it may be used on dry, mature skin to stimulate activity in sebaceous glands, but this must only be done for a short time (4–5 minutes).
- The treatment time for oily skin is 10–15 minutes.

THE INDIRECT METHOD

- With the indirect method, the current is carried to the client via a saturator electrode which is held in the client's hand. The current is then 'drawn off' through the fingers of the therapist massaging the skin. The therapist forms part of the circuit for the indirect method.
- It is used for its warming and relaxing effect.
- Skin types that benefit from indirect high frequency are: dry, dehydrated skin; sluggish skin; mature, tired skin with fine lines.
- The treatment time is 8–20 minutes depending upon the skin type and client tolerance.

DANGERS OF HIGH FREQUENCY TREATMENTS

- Shock because of the easy discharge of the current. Ensure that the client removes all metal jewellery and that she cannot accidentally touch metal objects, such as trolleys and bed frames.
- The destruction of tissues through sparking when using the direct method. Sparking must be done quickly over a pustule with less than a 7 mm gap ($\frac{1}{4}$ in).

QUESTIONS

1 Explain what is meant by a high frequency current.

2 Give two different methods of application.

3 List the skin types which would benefit from each method.

4 Explain what is meant by 'sparking'.

5 When would sparking be used and at what distance?

6 How does sparking produce its effect?

7 List the contra-indications to direct high frequency treatment.

8 Explain why the electrode must be and remain in contact with the skin when the current is switched on and off.

9 Which method is most suitable for the tense client with mature, dry skin?

10 Why is the therapist said to be part of the circuit in the indirect method?

11 Give the main dangers to the client when using high frequency treatment.

12 Explain the procedure for cleaning the electrodes after use.

CHAPTER 3

Mechanical massage

Figure 3.1   *A gyratory massager*

Figure 3.1 is a photograph of just one type of equipment used for mechanical massage. Mechanical massage is the manipulation of body tissues using machines. Generally, mechanical massage is used in conjunction with other treatments to relieve muscle tension and muscle pain, to improve the circulation and to improve certain skin conditions. Providing the client is on a reducing diet, the heavier vibrations may help to disperse fatty deposits from specific areas of the body.

Many different types of appliances are manufactured to produce effects similar to those of a manual massage. They vary from the small hand-held percussion and audio-sonic equipment designed to treat small, localised areas, to the large heavy gyratory vibrators used for deeper effects on large areas of the body. Although the effects are similar to those of manual massage, the sensation felt by the client is very different. The treatment is rather impersonal and the use of a machine rather than the touch of hands is not as pleasing to the client.

In practice, most mechanical vibratory treatments should be combined with some manual massage, thus gaining the more personal aspects of manual massage combined with the depth and power of vibratory equipment. Using mechanical massage equipment is certainly less tiring for the beauty therapist than performing a long, vigorous manual massage. The effects produced are similar for all types of massage equipment, but are deeper and greater with the heavier machines. The treatment is very popular with clients as they feel invigorated and consider that the desired results will be achieved.

Gyratory vibrator

Massage with this type of appliance is much heavier than with percussion and audio-sonic vibrators. It is therefore more suitable for heavier work on large and bulky areas of the body. There are two main types of appliance.

Figure 3.2   *A hand-held massager*

1 *The hand-held vibrator.* This is heavy to use as all the electrical component parts are held in the hand. It is useful for domicillary work.
2 *The floor-standing vibrator commonly called G5.* This is a very popular treatment in the salon. Here all the electrical components are housed in a box which is supported by a stand, and only the moving head is held in the hand. This machine uses a rotary electric motor to turn a crank, which is attached to the head. The head is driven to turn in gyratory motion, moving round and round, up and down and side to side with pressure, providing a deep massage. A variety of attachments is available, which screw on to the head; they are designed to simulate the movements of manual massage:
   (a) Effleurage: sponge heads, curved and disc.
   (b) Petrissage: hard rubber heads, single and double ball, flat disc, four half-ball (egg box), multi-hard spike.
   (c) Tapotement: fine spiky and brush heads.

Figure 3.3   *Examples of different heads for the gyratory massager*

USES

1 For spot reduction of fatty deposits in conjunction with other treatments and reduced food intake.
2 To relieve muscular tension.
3 To reduce muscular aches and pains.
4 To improve poor circulation.
5 To improve the texture of dry, flaky, rough skin.

EFFECTS

1 As with manual massage, the main effect is stimulation of the circulation. The movements speed up the flow of blood in the veins, removing de-oxygenated blood and waste products more rapidly. This affects the arterial circulation bringing oxygenated blood and nutrients to the area. Lymph drainage via the lymphatic vessels is also increased.
2 Increased blood supply will increase the metabolic rate in the tissues. This will improve the condition of the tissues.
3 Increased blood supply and friction of the heads will raise the temperature of the area, thus will aid muscle relaxation and relieve pain.
4 Pain in muscles may also be relieved due to rapid removal of waste products, such as lactic acid.
5 Surface capillaries dilate giving an erythema. This improves skin tone.
6 The desquamating effect of the heads may improve the texture of the skin.
7 The continuous heavy pressure on adipose tissue and increased circulation to the area may aid the dispersion of fatty deposits if the client is on a reducing diet.

CONTRA-INDICATIONS

1 Skin diseases and disorders.
2 Bruises.
3 Dilated capillaries.
4 Varicose veins.
5 Thrombosis or phlebitis.
6 Skin tags, warts or pigmented moles.
7 Recent operations and scar tissue.
8 Treatment of the abdomen during pregnancy and menstruation.
9 Extremely hairy areas.
10 Thin, bony clients.
11 Elderly clients with thin, crêpy skin and lack of subcutaneous fat.
12 Acute back and spinal problems, eg disc trouble.

DANGERS

Heavy and prolonged treatments can cause bruising and dilated capillaries.

PRECAUTIONS

1 Check for contra-indications.
2 Do not use heavy percussion over bony areas or over the abdomen with poor muscle tone.
3 Do not over treat one area, keep the head moving.
4 Keep the head surface parallel to the surface of the body and adapt to body contours.
5 Hold the head away from the client when switching on in case the head is insecure and becomes detached. Hold the head below the bed for safety.
6 Cover the heads with a plastic bag, which can be changed for each client, for hygienic reasons.

Figure 3.4 *Demonstration of treatment using gyratory massager*

TREATMENT TECHNIQUE

PREPARATION OF THE CLIENT

1 Place the client in a well-supported comfortable position.
2 Check that all jewellery has been removed.
3 Check for contra-indications.
4 Clean the skin with cologne.
5 Explain the treatment to the client.
6 Select the appropriate pre-heating treatment.
7 Apply talc to the area using effleurage strokes (do not use oil as it may cause deterioration of the sponge heads).

PROCEDURE

I Select the appropriate heads to suit the needs of the client. Do not change the heads too often as this breaks the continuity of the treatment:

(a) For effleurage: curved sponge on limbs or round sponge elsewhere.

(b) For kneading: the flat disc head for lighter petrissage; the four ball head for deeper petrissage; the multi, large spike for very deep petrissage on very heavy areas of adipose tissue; single and double ball heads on specific, localised areas.

(c) For desquamating: fine spiky and brush heads.

To maintain high standards of hygiene, the heads can be placed in a plastic bag, which should be changed for each client.

2 Switch the machine on holding the head below the level of the couch. (This is a safety precaution in case the head is insecure – if it flies off it will not hit the client).

3 With the sponge applicator, apply in long sweeping strokes following the direction of venous return and natural contours of the body. The stroke at make and break should be light and smooth rather than abrupt and jerky. The pressure should be heavier on muscle bulk. Cover the area well.

4 Change the head for kneading. Use a circular kneading motion, using the other hand to support the tissues and lift them towards the head. Again apply upward pressure and work with venous return. Cover the area well.

5 Keep the surface of the attachment parallel to the surface of the body at all times. (If one side lifts off the body, there is a danger of damaging the tissues with the hard edge of the head.)

6 Change to the effleurage head to complete the treatment.

7 The degree of erythema and client tolerance dictates the length of the treatment.

8 Wash the heads in hot water and detergent, and allow them to dry.

Note: Particular care should be taken when selecting heads for treating the abdominal wall. Abdominal organs have no bony framework for protection – their only protection is provided by the muscles and tissues of the abdominal wall. Over-stretched muscles with poor tone offer less protection. This must be considered when treating the abdomen. The heavier petrissage heads should only be used on well-toned abdominal muscles with a covering of adipose tissue, eg the younger, overweight client.

Figure 3.5a and b   *Direction of strokes for gyratory massager*

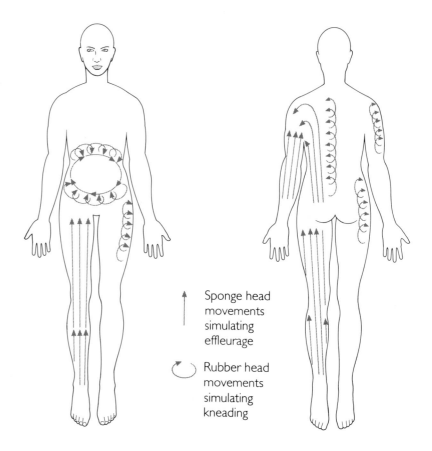

↑ Sponge head movements simulating effleurage

↻ Rubber head movements simulating kneading

Head
Switch
Adjustment knob

Figure 3.6   *Percussion vibrator*

Percussion vibrator

This is a hand-held appliance; it is lightweight, easy to use and to transport. As its name suggests, it is similar in effect to manual percussion movements. An electric motor is used to make the head move or tap up and down on the skin. The head can be fitted with a variety of attachments, eg sponge or spike. Some percussion vibrators have an adjustment knob for increasing and decreasing the intensity of the tap. As the knob is tightened, the tap intensity decreases; as the knob is released the tap intensity increases. This should be carefully controlled to suit the tissues being treated. The number of movements per second is constant relating to the frequency of the current. With mains frequency of 50 Hz (cycles per second), each tap occurs every half cycle, therefore the rate of tapping will be 100 per second. Treatment time may vary from 5–15 minutes depending on the desired effects. It is used mainly on the face, neck and across the shoulders.

USES

1 To stimulate dry, dehydrated or mature skin. The improved circulation and increase in metabolic rate will improve the condition of the skin.
2 To stimulate sebaceous glands; the warmth generated in the tissues will stimulate the production and release of sebum, which will help to lubricate the dry, tired, mature skin.
3 To aid desquamation of a sluggish skin, the friction of the heads on the body part will aid the removal of the surface layer, improving texture of the skin.
4 To improve and maintain the condition of normal skin.
5 To promote relaxation of muscle fibres, the warmth produced in the area will aid relaxation and relieve tension. It is particularly effective over localised tension nodules.

EFFECTS

1 An increase in circulation to the treated area, bringing nutrients and oxygen to the area and removing waste products. This improves the condition of the tissues.
2 It produces vasodilation, giving hyperaemia and erythema, improving the colour and tone of the skin.
3 It increases the metabolic rate, thus improving the condition of the tissues.
4 The increase in circulation and the friction of the heads raises the temperature of the area. This promotes relaxation, relieves pain and may stimulate the activity of sebaceous glands.
5 The friction of the heads aids desquamation; this removes the surface layer of cells, improving the condition of the skin.

CONTRA-INDICATIONS

1 Any skin diseases or inflammatory disorders.
2 Infected acne.
3 Highly vascular or telangiectic skin or dilated capillaries.
4 Sinus problems.
5 Headaches or migraines.
6 Lean bony features.
7 Mature skin with poor elasticity.

PRECAUTIONS

1 Check for contra-indications.
2 Do not use over very bony areas.
3 Avoid the eye region.

4 Keep the head surface parallel to the surface of the face.
5 Do not over treat one area – keep the head moving.

Audio-sonic vibrator

This is another type of hand-held appliance. Its name is derived from the fact that the machine produces a humming sound (it should not be confused with ultra-sound therapy, which is quite different). This vibrator uses an electromagnet. When the current is passing one way, the coil moves forward; as the current reverses, the coil moves back. This movement forward and backward is transmitted to the head of the appliance. When the head is placed on the tissues, the forward-backward movement of the coil alternately compress and decompress the tissues. Because the head does not physically move forward and backward, this appliance has a gentler action than the percussion vibrator. It penetrates more deeply into the tissues, but is less stimulating on the surface of the skin. It is, therefore, more suitable for use on sensitive areas of the face and on a mature skin. It is particularly useful for relaxing tension nodules.

Figure 3.7   *Audio-sonic vibrator*

Adjustment knob

Head

Switch

USES

Similar to the percussion vibrator.

1 To generally improve the condition of sensitive skin.
2 To stimulate the dry, dehydrated, mature skin.
3 To stimulate the sallow skin.
4 To aid desquamation and improve sluggish skin.
5 To produce warmth and aid relaxation of muscle fibres. Particularly effective over tension nodules.

EFFECTS

Similar to the percussion vibrator:

1 An increase in circulation.
2 It produces vasodilation.
3 It increases the metabolic rate.
4 It raises the temperature, therefore promotes relaxation of muscle fibres and stimulates activity of sebaceous glands.
5 It aids desquamation.

CONTRA-INDICATIONS AND PRECAUTIONS

See 'Percussion vibrator'.

TREATMENT TECHNIQUE FOR PERCUSSION AND AUDIO-SONIC VIBRATORS

PREPARATION OF THE CLIENT

1 Place the client in a well-supported and comfortable position.
2 Check that all jewellery has been removed.
3 Check for contra-indications.
4 Explain the treatment to the client.
5 Cleanse the skin.
6 Apply talc for oily/normal skin or cream for dry skin. (Read the manufacturer's instructions.)

PROCEDURE

1 Select the appropriate head and secure it firmly to the vibrator.
2 Switch the machine on away from the client.
3 Commence the treatment using straight lines or a circular motion; ensure coverage of all areas, but avoid delicate areas around the eyes and prominent cheek-bones.
4 The skin reaction indicates the length of the treatment time. When an even erythema is produced, the treatment should stop. This may take between 5–15 minutes.
5 The vibrator can be used indirectly over bony or sensitive areas, eg cheek-bones and forehead. The therapist places her hand between the face and the vibrator head. This reduces the stimulation.
6 Remove the talc or cream and complete the facial routine.
7 Clean the heads, wash with hot water and detergent and disinfect with surgical wipes. Brushes and sponges may be soaked in disinfectant.

Belt massager

These are usually made of canvas strapping; some have small, ball-like studding in the strapping. The belt is positioned around the area to be treated and the motor moves it back and forth with vibratory motion.

It is generally used to aid the dispersal of fat (providing the client is on a diet) around the waist, hips and thighs.

SUMMARY

- Mechanical massage is the manipulation of body tissues using machines.
- Types of mechanical massage equipment: gyratory vibrators – hand-held and floor-standing models; percussion vibrators; audio-sonic massagers; belt massagers.
- The hand-held vibrators are used for small body and facial areas; the large vibrators are used on large body areas.
- Mechanical massage is used to improve many conditions. It is usually combined with some manual massage. The client will then benefit from the personal touch and from the deeper effect of the mechanical massage.
- Mechanical massage will improve the circulation to the area, will relieve muscle tension and aches and pains, will aid the dispersal of fatty tissue in conjunction with diet and will improve the condition of the skin.
- There is little danger in application except that bruising and dilated capillaries may result from heavy or prolonged treatment.
- The vibrator head moves round and round with gyratory movement. It is used on the body.
- The percussion vibrator head moves up and down and taps on the body part. It is used on small areas, such as tension nodules, or on the face to improve the condition of the skin.
- The audio-sonic vibrator alternately compresses and decompresses the tissues due to the movement of an electromagnet within the head. Because the head does not physically tap on the area, it is much more gentle in action than the percussion vibrator. It is used on painful tension nodules and on the face to improve the condition of the skin; it is particularly suitable for sensitive skins.
- The belt massager moves back and forth with vibratory action. It is used to aid dispersal of fatty deposits providing the client is on a diet.

QUESTIONS

1 Give three uses for mechanical massage on the body.

2 Name three different types of mechanical massage equipment.

3 List four contra-indications to mechanical massage on the body.

4 List the effects of mechanical massage on the body.

5 Explain briefly why audio-sonic vibrators have an advantage over percussion vibrators on a sensitive area.

6 Give four effects of percussion vibrator treatment to the face.

7 Give two different uses for each of the following:
  (a) gyratory vibrator (G5).
  (b) percussion vibrator.
  (c) audio-sonic vibrator.

8 Explain briefly how you would incorporate mechanical massage into a body treatment routine.

9 Give reasons why the heavy gyratory vibrator heads should not be used on the abdominal wall of certain clients.

10 Explain the procedure for maintaining high standards of hygiene when using gyratory vibrators.

CHAPTER 4

Vacuum suction

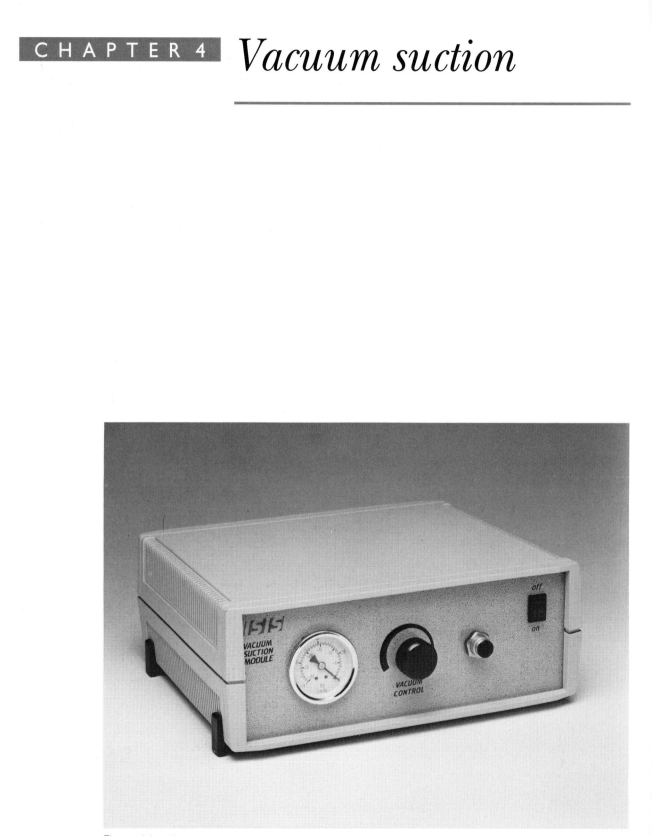

Figure 4.1 *A vacuum suction machine used for facial and body work.*

OBJECTIVES

After you have studied this chapter you will be able to:

1 Identify the terminals on the machine.
2 Describe the lymphatic system.
3 Draw outlines of the face and body and indicate the positions of the main lymph nodes relevant to lymphatic drainage.
4 Identify the main lymph nodes on the human body.
5 Determine the suitability of the treatment to meet the needs of the client.
6 Describe the effects of facial and body vacuum suction.
7 Identify the contra-indications to treatment.
8 Treat the client paying due consideration to maximum efficiency, comfort, safety and hygiene.

Figure 4.1 is a photograph of a vacuum suction machine. This particular model may be used for both facial and body work, and includes a variety of cups called ventouse to suit different areas of the body. It is used to speed up the flow of lymph and blood and stimulate the metabolic rate. The treatment is based on the principle of creating reduced pressure within the cups. These are moved over the area in the direction of lymphatic drainage towards the nearest lymph nodes, into which the lymph will drain. When the pressure within the cup is reduced to below atmospheric pressure, the tissues rise into the cup. The lymphatic and blood vessels dilate as the suction is applied, and as the cup moves along the rate of flow will increase. Vacuum suction treatment is effective on the face and the body.

The lymphatic system

In order to provide the most effective treatment, the therapist must have an understanding of the lymphatic system. The lymphatic system is closely associated with the blood circulatory system. It transports a fluid called lymph from the tissue spaces, and returns it to the blood via the subclavian veins. If this fluid is not drained away from tissue spaces, swelling of the area will occur – this is known as oedema.

Lymphatic capillaries begin as blind end tubes and form a network throughout the tissue spaces. Their walls are very thin, allowing particles of large molecular size to pass through.

Large protein molecules and waste products are transported via the lymphatic system. Lymph capillaries join together to form larger vessels. These lymph vessels are similar to small veins in structure and have semi-lunar valves lining their walls to prevent the backward flow of lymph. All lymph vessels drain into lymph nodes. These are small, bean-shaped structures strategically placed in groups throughout the body. The lymph is filtered as it passes through each node; damaged cells, microbes, etc, are filtered and destroyed. In the nodes, lymphocytes multiply and antibodies are produced; these may be carried via the lymph into the circulation. After leaving the nodes, the lymphatic vessels join to form even larger lymph trunks. These empty into one of two lymphatic ducts:

1   *The thoracic duct* drains the whole of the body apart from the upper right quarter; it empties into the left subclavian vein.
2   *The right lymphatic duct* drains the right arm, right side of the head and chest; it empties into the right subclavian vein.

The speed at which lymph flows through the system depends on many factors. The contraction and relaxation of muscles help its return, as does the negative pressure and movement of the chest during respiration. Backward flow of lymph is prevented by valves in the vessel walls. The volume of lymph passing into the capillaries depends on the arterial pressure and pressure of the tissue fluid.

During vacuum suction treatment, it is essential to follow the course of the lymphatic vessels and end at the nearest set of lymph nodes.

Figure 4.2   *The structure of a lymph node*

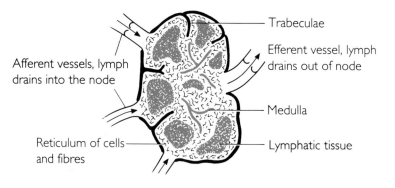

Afferent vessels, lymph drains into the node

Reticulum of cells and fibres

Trabeculae

Efferent vessel, lymph drains out of node

Medulla

Lymphatic tissue

Table 4.1 *Nodes of the body and face*

Body nodes	Facial nodes
Axillary nodes (in armpit)	Superficial cervical
Supratrochlear nodes (at elbow)	Deep cervical
Supraclavicular (above clavicle)	Parotid
Inguinal nodes (in groin)	Buccal
Popliteal nodes (behind knee)	Submandibular
	Submental
	Post-auricular (mastoid)
	Occipital

Vacuum suction units

Some of these are designed as facial units, some as body units, while others are combined units for the treatment of the face and body (see Figure 4.1). They all consist of a machine, and a selection of cups or ventouse which connect to it by plastic tubing. A suction effect is produced in the cups by sucking out air to reduce the pressure. This is done using a vacuum pump driven by an electric motor. The amount of negative pressure is registered on a gauge, and can be controlled by increasing or decreasing a regulating knob. The on/off switch controls the power from the mains. Most machines have a second outlet for blowing the air out – this can be used as a spray for a variety of preparations.

The cups are manufactured in various sizes and shapes to suit the areas of the body to be treated: small cups are for facial work and large cups are for body work. The selection of the appropriate cup to suit the body part must be carefully considered. Cups are made of glass, plastic or metal. Some cups have a small hole in the side to release the vacuum when required. This hole must be covered with a finger to maintain a vacuum (the finger is removed to release the vacuum). If there is no hole, the vacuum must be released by depressing the flesh with the finger.

Facial vacuum suction

Vacuum suction may be used on the face and neck for general cleansing on normal, dry combination and greasy skins. It can be used to loosen blocked pores and black heads (comedones) and to improve the condition of dry, dehydrated skin.

Figure 4.3   *Small vacuum suction machine showing facial and body cups*

USES

1 General skin cleansing on normal, dry, combination and greasy skins. This can be carried out following steam treatment. The time for the cleansing treatment is 5 minutes.
2 The deep cleansing of seborrhoeic skin to remove dead keratinised cells and sebum and clear follicular blockages. This is most effective following steam or disincrustation treatments to the face. The time for the treatment is 10–12 minutes.
3 To stimulate dry, dehydrated skins and improve their condition. The increased circulation, increased removal of waste products and increased cellular activity will all contribute to the improvement of the skin. The time for the treatment is 10–12 minutes.

EFFECTS

1 It speeds up the removal of waste products via the lymphatic system.
2 It increases blood circulation to the area, bringing nutrients and oxygen thus improving the condition of the skin.
3 It produces vasodilation giving an erythema and improving skin tone.
4 It stimulates cell metabolism.
5 It aids desquamation and the removal of dead keratinised cells, and improves the texture of the skin.
6 It loosens blockages and comedones, cleansing the pores.

CONTRA-INDICATIONS

1 Areas of telangiectasis.
2 Delicate sensitive skin.
3 Loose crêpy skin, eg around eyes.
4 Areas of thin skin and fine texture.
5 Infected acne.
6 Skin disorders/diseases.
7 Sun burnt or wind burnt skin.

PRECAUTIONS

1 Select the correct cup to suit the area.
2 Check the pressure on yourself, and adjust the pressure to suit the flesh on the area being treated.
3 Apply sufficient oil to the area to facilitate the movement of the cup and provide a seal.
4 Lift enough flesh – do not exceed 20 per cent of the cup.

5 Lift the cup and move it across the contours of the face to the nearest set of lymph nodes. Do not work over the nodes.

6 Release the pressure before lifting the cup off the area.

7 Overlap the previous stroke.

8 Do not over treat the area.

9 Speak to the client during the treatment.

Figure 4.4   *Facial vacuum suction treatment*

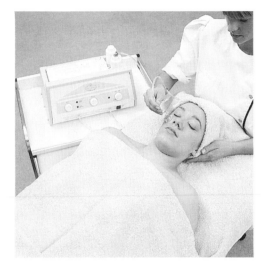

TREATMENT TECHNIQUE

PREPARATION OF THE CLIENT

1 Place the client in a well-supported and comfortable position.

2 Check that all jewellery has been removed.

3 Check for contra-indications.

4 Explain the treatment to the client.

5 Cleanse the skin, apply steam or disincrustation treatment.

6 Apply oil to the face and neck.

PROCEDURE

1 Place the machine on a stable base and check the plug and leads.

2 Check that the intensity controls are at zero.

3 Collect all commodities.

4 Test the machine.

5 Wipe the cup with disinfecting fluid, eg surgical spirit.

6 Select the appropriate cup.

7 Place the cup on the area and adjust the suction – do not exceed 20 per cent of the ventouse. Hold it like a pencil and perpendicular to the skin.

8 Lift the cup and glide it according to the contours of the face to the nearest set of lymph nodes.

9 Break the suction before lifting the cup off the skin (use the release hole or depress the skin with the little finger).

10 Move on to the next stroke; overlap the previous stroke until the area is covered. Repeat 5–8 times depending upon the skin reaction and whether the skin is pre-heated. An erythema will develop more quickly if the skin is preheated.

11 Continue until the neck and face are covered. The pattern of strokes on page 58 is a guideline of the drainage to named nodes.

12 Use the appropriate cup for extracting comedones and blockages or for treating wrinkles.

13 Remove the oil and tone.

14 Wash the cup and tube in hot water and detergent and sterilise by soaking in disinfectant such as Milton, Cydex or Barbicide.

Figure 4.5   *Lymphatic nodes of the face and neck*

Figure 4.6   *Direction of strokes for facial vacuum suction*

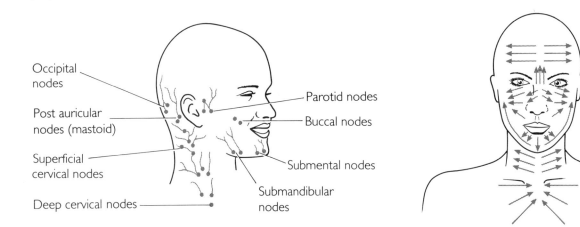

Occipital nodes

Post auricular nodes (mastoid)

Superficial cervical nodes

Deep cervical nodes

Parotid nodes

Buccal nodes

Submental nodes

Submandibular nodes

Body vacuum suction

Vacuum suction on the body is always used in conjunction with other treatments. The suction may be applied by the moving cup method or may be applied using stationary cups with a pulsating on-off vacuum.

USES

1 To reduce fatty deposits on the abdomen, hips, thighs, dowager's hump below the neck, etc, in conjunction with other treatments and diet.

2 To improve and reduce areas of cellulite.

3 To improve poor circulation, both lymphatic and blood.

4 To reduce non-systemic oedema and areas of fluid retention.

5 To improve the condition of the skin.

EFFECTS

1 The flow of lymph is speeded up. As previously explained, the negative pressure inside the cup makes the tissues rise into the cup. As it does this, the vessels dilate and fill up with lymph; as the cup moves along it draws lymph with it as the vessels expand and recoil. The stroke will end just before the lymph node and lymph will drain into the node. As the flow of lymph is speeded up, more waste products will be removed.

2 Oedema may be reduced. Because the flow of lymph in the vessels is speeded up, more lymph will be drained from the tissues thus reducing stagnation and swelling. This works well for gravitational oedema but not for oedema caused by high blood pressure, kidney problems and other systemic problems. (Seek a doctor's advice to establish the cause of the oedema.)

3 Circulation is increased. In the same way as lymph vessels are affected, the veins will alternately expand and recoil and the venous flow is speeded up. If blood flows more quickly in the veins, then the arterial side will also speed up. This increases the supply of nutrients and oxygen to the body part and speeds up the removal of waste. This will improve the condition of the tissues.

4 The increased circulation will produce heat and vasodilation with erythema (this improves the colour of the skin).

5 Cell metabolism is stimulated and this improves the condition of the skin.

6 The friction of the cup, the oil used on the part and the stimulation of the circulation will aid desquamation, thus also improving the condition of the skin.

7 Venous flow is speeded up and this can help to prevent varicose veins. (If varicose veins are already present, do not use vacuum suction as it will exacerbate the condition.)

CONTRA-INDICATIONS

1 Skin diseases and disorders, sunburn.
2 Broken capillaries (thread veins) or varicose veins.
3 Recent stretch marks and scars.
4 Loose, crêpy skin and ageing thin skin.
5 Bruises.
6 Thin bony areas.
7 Very hairy areas.
8 Breast tissue.
9 Thrombosis.
10 Phlebitis.

DANGERS

1 Bruising of the area caused by poor technique. Bruising may be caused:
   (a) if the pressure is too high;
   (b) pulling the cup off before releasing the vacuum;
   (c) over-treating area with too many strokes or too long a treatment;
   (d) pushing the cup downwards instead of lifting and gliding.
2 Making thread veins worse if they are not avoided.
3 Over-stretching ageing, thin skin.

PRECAUTIONS

1 Select the correct size of cup to fit the area (the largest possible without losing suction).
2 Check the pressure on yourself.
3 Apply sufficient oil to the area to facilitate the movement of the cup and provide a seal.
4 Lift enough flesh, but do not exceed 20 per cent of the cup.
5 Lift the cup and move it in a straight line to the nearest set of lymph nodes. (Do not work over the nodes.)
6 Release pressure before lifting the cup off the area.
7 Overlap the previous stroke by 1 cm ($\frac{1}{2}$ in).
8 Do not over treat the area.

Figure 4.7 *Body vacuum suction treatment*

Treatment technique

PREPARATION OF THE CLIENT

1 Place the client in a well-supported and comfortable position.
2 Check that all jewellery has been removed.
3 Check for contra-indications.
4 Explain the treatment to the client.
5 Select the appropriate pre-heating treatment.
6 If the client has not taken a shower, clean the skin with cologne or surgical spirit.
7 Apply oil or cream to the area to facilitate the movement of the cup and to provide a seal between the cup and the skin.

PROCEDURE

1 Place the machine on a stable base and check the plug, leads and tube.
2 Check the intensity controls are at zero.
3 Collect all commodities.
4 Test the machine. (This may be done by placing a finger over the inlet hole and watching the dial, or by placing the cup on the forearm until suction is felt; this must then be adjusted to suit the flesh on the area being treated.)
5 Select cups of suitable size – the largest possible to fit the area without losing suction.
6 Wipe the cup with disinfectant wipes or surgical spirit swabs.
7 Place the cup on the area and adjust the suction so that the skin fills 20 per cent of the cup. (Break the suction quickly if suction is too high, otherwise bruising and dilation of capillaries may occur.)
8 Lift the cup and glide it in a straight line towards the nearest set of lymph nodes that drain the area.
Note: Pressing the cup down instead of lifting can be painful and may cause bruising.
9 Break the suction by removing finger from the hole on the cup. If there is no hole, depress the flesh with the little finger under the rim of the cup or use the thumb of the other hand to depress the flesh.
Note: The pressure must be released before the cup is lifted otherwise bruising and dilated capillaries may occur.
10 Move to the adjacent area overlapping the last stroke by 1 cm or $\frac{1}{2}$ in only. Continue until all the area is covered. Return over the first stroke and cover the area five to ten times depending on the type of flesh and desired effect.
Note: Do not repeat the stroke over the same area without moving on – this can cause dilated capillaries.

The rhythm should be of medium even speed, not too fast or too slow. The sequence should be as follows:

(a) place the cup on the body part, filling 20 per cent of the cup;

(b) lift the cup and move it in a straight line towards the nearest lymph nodes draining that area;

(c) release the pressure;

(d) the next stroke should overlap the last stroke by 1 cm or $\frac{1}{2}$ in if possible.

11 At the end of the treatment, effleurage the area and remove oil from the body part.

12 Clean the cups and tube – wash in hot water and detergent, dry and wipe with disinfectant wipes, or soak in disinfectant.

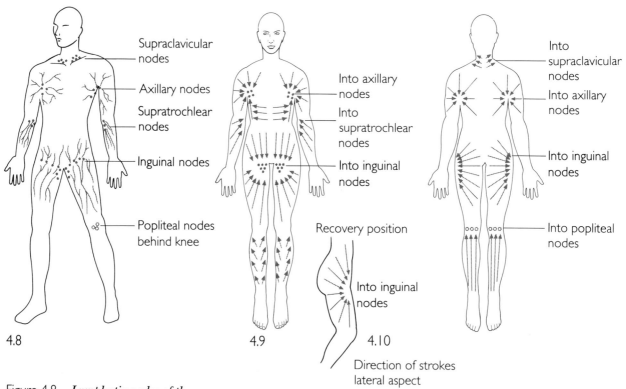

4.8

4.9

4.10

Direction of strokes lateral aspect

Figure 4.8 *Lymphatic nodes of the body*
Figure 4.9 *Direction of strokes (anterior aspect)*
Figure 4.10 *Direction of strokes (posterior and lateral aspect)*

Vacuum suction should form part of a treatment routine – pre-heating followed by gyratory vibrator or manual massage to warm and soften the area and increase circulation. This can be followed by vacuum suction then electrical muscle stimulation (EMS) or exercises.

If galvanic treatment has been given, do not use vacuum suction over the area of the pads as the skin will be very sensitive. Vacuum suction can be done prior to galvanic treatment to decongest the area.

Pulsating multi-cup vacuum suction

Multi-cup vacuum suction machines are manufactured for treating localised, large areas. They have the advantage of not requiring the constant effort of the therapist. However, care and practice is necessary to select the correct high and low pressure in each individual cup. This treatment is only suitable for obese clients with a considerable covering of adipose tissue.

MACHINES

These machines are similar to the single cup vacuum suction units, but are larger and have four to six outlets (each outlet has its own shut off valve). Plastic tubing connects the cups to the outlets. The cups come in various sizes and are selected to suit the area being treated. The reduced pressure created by these machines is always 'pulsed'. This allows for a period of high suction and a period of low suction. The high suction time must be carefully controlled to produce the required effect, but not so high that it damages capillaries causing bruising of tissues. The low suction period must be just high enough to keep the cup on the part, but it must allow the tissues to relax. Treatments should commence with longer periods of low suction. Periods of high suction should be gradually increased according to the client's tolerance.

Figure 4.11 *A vacuum suction machine used for facial and body treatments including pulsating action*

TREATMENT TECHNIQUE

PREPARATION OF THE CLIENT

Prepare the client as for gliding vacuum suction (see page 61).

PROCEDURE

1 Place the machine on a suitable stable base and check the plugs and leads are secure.
2 Check that the intensity controls are at zero.
3 Collect all commodities.
4 Test the machine.
5 Commence treatment with a gliding method to introduce the treatment to client.
6 Position the first cup, open its valve, adjust the main control until the required 'lift' of flesh is obtained, switch on the pulse rhythm and adjust the control so that the flesh relaxes, but the cup does not fall off.
7 Repeat this for all the cups.
8 Adjust the pulse to alter the length and degree of 'lift' if necessary.
9 Slide the cups to a new area at regular intervals to prevent over-treating and bruising.
10 At the end of the treatment, switch off each valve in turn and remove the cups.
11 Use a gliding single-cup method to drain the area for around 5 minutes at the end of the treatment. Pulsating treatments can be applied for 10–15 minutes depending on the client's skin reaction and tolerance.
12 Wash all the cups and tubes with hot water and detergent, dry and wipe over with disinfectant wipes, or soak them in disinfectant.

SUMMARY

- This treatment speeds up the flow of lymph in the lymphatic vessels and, therefore, removes waste products from the area more quickly and reduces any oedema in the area. It also increases the circulation to the area, bringing oxygen and nutrients to the body part and removing waste products.

THE LYMPHATIC SYSTEM

- Small blind end tubes, called lymphatic capillaries, form a network through tissue spaces between cells; they join to form larger lymphatic vessels. These vessels drain into lymph nodes where lymph is filtered; lymph nodes also produce lymphocytes. Afferent lymph vessels enter the nodes; efferent lymph vessels leave the nodes. Lymph vessels eventually form lymph trunks which drain into the thoracic duct or into the right lymphatic duct and then into the right and left subclavian veins.

lymph from tissue spaces	→	lymph capillaries	→	lymph vessels	→	lymph nodes	→	lymph trunks	→ thoracic duct →	subclavian veins
									→ right lymphatic duct →	

Table F *The main lymph nodes of the face and body*

Facial Nodes	**Body Nodes**
Superficial cervical	Axillary nodes (in the armpit or
Deep cervical	axilla)
	Inguinal nodes (in the groin)
Mastoid	Supratrochlear nodes (at the
Parotid	elbow)
Buccal	Popliteal nodes (behind the knee)
Submental	Supraclavicular nodes (above the
Submandibular	clavicle – it drains the dowager's
Occipital	hump region).

- Vacuum suction on the face is used for general and deep cleansing and to stimulate and improve the condition of the dry, dehydrated skin.
- The treatment time for general cleansing is 5 minutes.
- The treatment time for deep cleansing is 10–12 minutes.
- The treatment time to improve condition of skin is 10–12 minutes.
- The above timings depend on the skin reaction.
- Vacuum suction is used on the body in conjunction with other treatments to improve the circulation of the blood and lymph, to aid dispersal of fatty deposits for clients on a diet, to improve areas of cellulite, and to reduce oedema.
- The treatment time will depend on the size of the area to be treated – the larger the area the longer the time needed to cover it (five to ten times).
- The main danger is causing bruising of the area. Bruising may be caused if the pressure is too high; by pulling the cup off before releasing the vacuum; by over-treating the area with too

many strokes; by pushing the cup down instead of lifting and gliding it.

● Other dangers are making thread veins worse and overstretching ageing skin.

QUESTIONS

1 Explain why the treatment is called vacuum suction.

2 Briefly explain how lymph is carried from the tissue spaces to the right and left subclavian veins.

3 Give two functions of lymph nodes and list the main nodes of the face and body.

4 What is meant by 'oedema'?

5 Give six contra-indications to facial vacuum suction treatment.

6 Explain the benefits of using vacuum suction on the face.

7 What prior treatment might be used to enhance the effect of vacuum suction to the face?

8 Give three reasons for using vacuum suction on the body.

9 How may the vacuum be released at the end of each stroke?

10 What is the purpose of applying oil to the area?

11 List three dangers associated with vacuum suction treatment.

12 How much flesh should be lifted into the cup?

13 How may bruising be caused in the area of application?

14 Explain how the cups and tubes should be dealt with after treatment, to ensure high standards of hygiene.

CHAPTER 5

Muscle stimulation

Figure 5.1 *Electronic machine for muscle stimulation*

After you have studied this chapter you will be able to:

1 Describe the structure of skeletal muscle tissue.
2 List the parts of the nervous system.
3 Differentiate between sensory, motor and connector neurones.
4 Explain the nature and transmission of a nerve impulse.
5 Describe the 'motor unit'.
6 Draw a diagram to illustrate the pathway of an impulse from the brain to a muscle fibre.
7 Differentiate between muscle fibre types and their stimulation by specific frequencies.
8 Describe the type of current and wave forms used for muscle stimulation.
9 List the factors that influence the response of the muscle.
10 Identify the position of the motor points of the superficial muscles of the body.
11 Explain the *three* different methods of padding.
12 Select suitable patterns of padding to suit the needs of the client.
13 Identify the controls on the machine and explain their effects.
14 Identify the contra-indications to treatment.
15 Apply pads accurately and securely to the body.
16 Select the appropriate parameters to suit the needs of the client.
17 Treat the client paying due consideration to maximum efficiency, comfort, safety and hygiene.

Figure 5.1 is a photograph of a modern, sophisticated electronic machine used for muscle stimulation. A variety of muscle stimulators are to be found on the market, and they range from simple single outlet machines with pre-set controls to the very complex machines with multi-outlets and a range of variable controls. However, they all produce electrical pulses which are applied to the body by means of electrodes. When the pulses are applied, they stimulate the motor nerves and result in the contraction of muscles. The muscles are made to contract and relax simulating active exercise. The treatment is used to improve muscle tone and condition and to maintain muscle strength.

Terminology of muscle contraction

Electrical impulses can be used to stimulate motor nerves and produce contraction of muscles. The impulses are produced by modifying direct or alternating currents. The current amplitude must be variable and must be of sufficient intensity and duration to produce a contraction.

Normal muscle contraction is brought about when impulses from the brain are transmitted via motor nerves to the muscles. The impulses produced by machines have the same effect as those from the brain. They stimulate the motor nerve directly and this will initiate a contraction in the muscles supplied by that nerve (see page 75).

The original current used for muscle stimulation was produced by the Smart-Bristow coil and was known as the *faradic current*. This term is sometimes used today to describe muscle stimulating treatments, eg faradism or faradic treatment. Manufacturers' names are also used to describe the treatments, eg Ultratone, Slendertone, Slim-line and others. The terms TENS, EMS and NMES (NMS) are also used.

- TENS means transcutaneous electrical nerve stimulation. This type of stimulation is used for pain control and is not generally used in beauty therapy. Modern equipment may include TENS to reduce pain and therefore improve client comfort.
- EMS means electrical muscle stimulation. This term covers stimulation of both innervated muscle and denervated muscle – innervated muscle refers to muscle with an intact nerve supply whilst denervated muscle means one lacking in nerve supply due to injury or disease. Different types of pulses are used for these two types of muscle.
- NMES or NMS means neuro-muscular (electrical) stimulation. This term covers the stimulation of innervated muscle. The pulse is used to stimulate a nerve and the impulse is transmitted via the nerve to the muscle, initiating a contraction.

Stimulation treatments in beauty therapy always use nerve stimulation to produce muscle contraction. Therefore, it is more accurate to use the terms NMES or NMS when referring to these treatments. However, EMS is commonly used.

Nerve-muscle physiology

In order to understand the action of muscle-stimulating currents, it is necessary to understand nerve-muscle function. The voluntary contraction of skeletal muscle is controlled by the brain. Impulses initiated in the brain are transmitted via the spinal cord and peripheral motor nerve to the muscle fibres, causing them to contract.

SKELETAL MUSCLE

Skeletal muscle is composed of long, thin, multinucleated cells called muscle fibres. These muscle fibres are composed of myofibrils separated by sarcoplasm, and they have an outer membrane called the sarcolemma. Muscle fibres are grouped together to form muscle bundles, and many bundles make up the complete muscle. Under an electron microscope, light and dark bands can be seen along the length of the fibre; these are known as A and I bands and are composed of two types of protein, actin and myosin. The movement of these bands into each other constitutes muscle contraction.

Figure 5.2   *Relaxed and contracted muscle fibres*

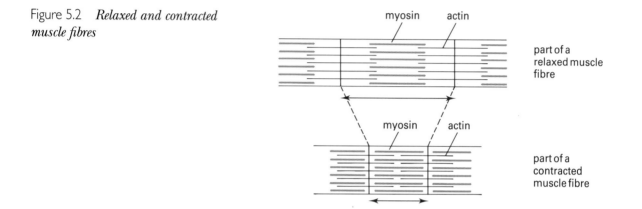

Muscles will contract in response to stimuli. Normally, these stimuli originate in the brain and are transmitted to muscle fibres via nerves. Because the stimuli are electrical in nature, a suitable electrical pulse from a machine can be used to initiate a contraction. The electrical pulse can be applied anywhere along the course of a motor nerve, but the best response is obtained if it is applied at the point where the nerve enters the belly of the muscle, known as the motor point. Each muscle fibre is sensitive to impulses reaching it from the central nervous system.

THE NERVOUS SYSTEM

The system is made up of:

1 The central nervous system comprising the brain and the spinal cord.
2 The peripheral nervous system comprising:
   (a) 12 pairs of cranial nerves arising from the brain;
   (b) 31 pairs of spinal nerves arising from the spinal cord.
3 The autonomic system.

Nervous tissue is composed of the functional units which conduct impulses, called *neurones,* and the supporting tissue, called *neuroglia.* There are three types of neurones:

1 Sensory neurones (or nerves): these carry impulses from the sensory organs to the spinal cord and brain.
2 Motor neurones: these carry impulses away from the brain and spinal cord to muscles and glands.
3 Connector neurones or interneurones: these are found in the brain and spinal cord and connect one group of neurones to another.

Neurones are similar in structure having a cell body and two types of processes called axons and dendrons.

● Axons carry impulses *away* from the cell body.
● Dendrons carry impulses *towards* the cell body.
● Dendrons have small terminal branches called *dendrites*.

Figure 5.3   *Types of neurones*
(a) Motor neurone (multipolar)
(b) Sensory neurone (unipolar)
(c) Interneurone (stellate)

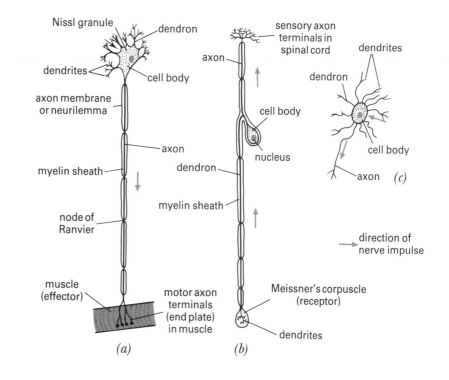

THE TRANSMISSION OF NERVE IMPULSES

Impulses are transmitted in axons and dendrons in one direction only. Impulses move along a nerve because of a change in its electrically charged state. This is brought about by the movement of positive and negative ions across the nerve membrane.

When the nerve membrane is at rest, solutions of sodium chloride, potassium chloride and various proteins are found inside and outside the membrane. The salts ionise in solution giving sodium (+) ions and chloride (−) ions outside, with potassium (+) ions and chloride (−) ions inside together with non-diffusable anions, negative proteins inside the membrane which maintain the negative potential across the membrane.

When the nerve membrane is non-conductive, there are more positive ions outside and more negative ions inside. Therefore a potential difference exists across the membrane. In this state of rest, the nerve is said to be *polarised*.

When a stimulus is applied to the nerve the following reactions will occur: there will be a fall of potential difference across the membrane; the permeability of the membrane changes; the diffusable ions move across the membrane until the polarity is reversed, ie there will be more negative ions outside and more positive ions inside. The nerve is now said to be *depolarised*.

When the concentration of ions reaches a certain level, the positive sodium ions are 'pumped out' and the nerve returns to its resting state, ie is repolarised. This change of state occurs along the nerve and constitutes the passage of the impulse.

Figure 5.4   *Passage of a nerve impulse along an axon*

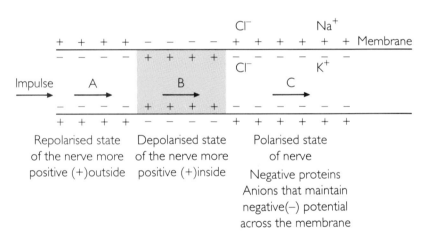

- The impulse leaves A and is transmitted to B when the polarity is reversed. The impulse will move along as the polarity returns to normal at B but reversed at C. The impulse is thus transmitted along the nerve fibre.
- More than one neurone will be involved in the transmission of a nerve impulse.
- Neurones do not connect directly with each other – there is always a gap between the end of one neurone and the beginning of another. This is known as a synapse.
- There are similar specialised synapses between motor neurones and muscle fibres known as the neuro-muscular junction. The impulse is transmitted across the gap by the chemical transmitter acetylcholine.

Figure 5.5   *Synapse between interconnecting neurones*

PATHWAY OF AN IMPULSE

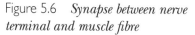

Figure 5.6   *Synapse between nerve terminal and muscle fibre*

Figure 5.7   *Motor nerve terminals stained with silver, and motor end plates stained with acetylcholinesterase*

An impulse initiated in the cells of the motor cortex of the brain will be transmitted via the axon (of the upper motor neurone) to the anterior/ventral horn of the spinal cord. Here the impulse will cross a synapse to stimulate the cell of another neurone (the lower motor neurone) to be transmitted via its axon to the muscle fibre.

Each anterior/ventral horn cell has one axon which leaves the spinal cord by the anterior/ventral root. The axons of many cells will emerge together as a motor nerve and pass to a muscle where they will enter at the *motor point*.

Each axon will then divide into many branches or terminals (from 5–150) depending on the function of the muscle. Muscles requiring fine control have smaller motor units with fewer branches and can, therefore, produce more finely graded movements.

Each axon branch will supply one muscle fibre. The junction between the axon branch and the muscle fibre is known as the neuro-muscular junction. Here the ends of the axons expand a little into bulbs; they approach but do not contact the muscle fibre. There is always a gap in between. The sarcolemma covering the muscle fibre is modified at this point and is known as the *motor end plate*.

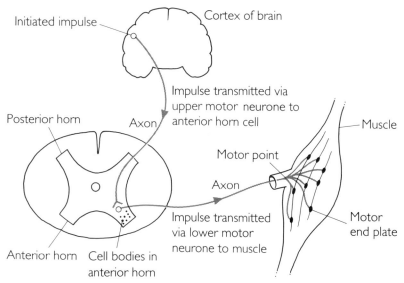

Figure 5.8   *Pathway of an impulse from the brain to a muscle fibre*

The anterior horn cell, the axon, axon branches and the muscle fibres they supply make up the *motor unit*. This is not only an anatomical unit but also a functional unit. Impulses generated at the anterior horn cell will pass via the axon to all the fibres supplied by the axon branches and all those fibres will contract simultaneously. The frequency of the impulses passing along the nerve will determine the strength of contraction in each motor unit.

During voluntary movement, motor units work an on/off 'shift' system. Some will contract while others will be at rest. When a stronger contraction is required, more motor units are activated. The frequency and number of motor units activated will determine the strength of contraction of the whole muscle.

Muscle fibre types

A muscle is composed of different types of muscle fibres. This enables individual muscles to perform various functions. Research has shown that these differences are imposed upon the fibres by their motor neurones. By imposing a certain pattern of activity on to the fibre, different physiological and biochemical properties develop. All the muscle fibres supplied by one motor neurone have similar properties.

Impulses from the central nervous system (CNS), which stimulate the different muscle fibres, are discharged at different frequencies (shown below). This becomes an important consideration when using electrical stimulation. Selection of the appropriate frequencies must be made for effective stimulation of the whole muscle. Specific frequencies can be used to produce certain characteristics in fibres when training athletes for particular events.

PROPERTIES OF MUSCLE FIBRES

- *Slow oxidative fibres (SO) red fibres or slow twitch fibres.* These fibres are capable of sustaining tension for long periods, and are active for nearly 24 hours per day. They have a high level of endurance without fatigue. Containing high levels of oxidative enzymes, they depend mainly on aerobic metabolism. They are well supplied with blood having a high-density capillary network. They are recruited for endurance activities, such as maintenance of posture, swimming and marathon running. Certain muscles will have a much higher proportion of these fibres, eg the soleus muscle. Impulses are transmitted to these fibres at frequencies of between 6 and 15 Hz.
- *Fast glycolytic fibres (FG) white fibres or fast twitch fibres.* These fibres are used intermittently for short periods only. They are

recruited when speed, eg reflex activity, and burst of power are required. They have low levels of endurance and fatigue easily. They have high levels of glycolytic enzymes and depend on anaerobic metabolism; they have a low-density capillary network. Certain muscles will have high proportions of these fibres, eg the orbital muscles of the eye, *orbicularis oculi*. Impulses are transmitted to these fibres at frequencies of between 30 and 80 Hz.

- *Fast oxidative glycolytic (FOG) fibres.* These are used for around 60 per cent of the day. They contain both oxidative and glycolytic enzymes and are recruited for general activities that require neither speed nor endurance. Impulses are transmitted to these fibres at frequencies of between 20 and 40 Hz.

A muscle will be composed of a mixture of fibres – the percentage of each fibre type will differ for each muscle and will depend on the function of the muscle. Research has shown that electrical stimulation can be used to change muscle properties.

If fast glycolytic muscle fibres are stimulated at frequencies between 6 and 15 Hz on a daily basis for a considerable length of time, they contract more slowly and do not fatigue easily. The biochemical characteristics are also changed; there is a decrease in glycolytic enzymes and an increase in oxidative enzymes; capillary density also increases. Thus fast glycolytic fibres can be changed to slow oxidative fibres (SO fibres do not respond in the same way).

This ability to change muscle fibre type is used medically (when a muscle has been transplanted and is required to change its function, eg replacing sphincters and cardiac assistance in heart disease).

Electrical stimulation

As explained above, a muscle will contract in response to an impulse from the brain, reaching it via its motor nerve. Stimuli or pulses of current produced by machines and applied to the motor nerve by electrodes will produce the same result, ie contraction of muscles supplied by that nerve.

Modern machines which produce these pulses are very sophisticated electronic units. (The older faradic current has now largely been replaced by interrupted direct current (see page 69)).

Some foreign units use modified AC, but British units in the main use modified DC. These units produce low frequency, interrupted direct current of between 10 and 120 Hz. There are units on the market which offer upper range low frequency current of between

200 and 800 Hz. Research has shown, however, that maximal force is developed in human muscle at between 40 and 80 Hz. There is, therefore, little purpose in using higher frequencies, and careful consideration should be given to the effects of using these frequencies. Although sensory stimulation is reduced by higher frequencies, and they 'feel more comfortable', their safety and some of the claims made should be questioned as the mode in which they work is unclear.

Although there is a large number of different units available, one basic concept remains common to all – impulses are produced which stimulate the motor nerves resulting in the contraction of muscles supplied by those nerves. The muscles are made to actively contract and then relax, improving their tone and condition and maintaining strength, providing that the treatment is carried out on a regular basis.

PULSES, IMPULSES AND STIMULI

- A constant flow of current or a slow, rising electrical pulse will not produce a contraction as the muscle adapts to the current. This is known as accommodation.
- The direct currrent must be modified to produce pulses which rise steeply and fall at regular intervals.
- The intensity must be high enough and the duration of the pulse long enough to produce a contraction.

Figure 5.9   *Sharp and slow rising pulses*

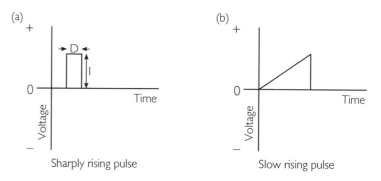

(a) Sharply rising pulse

(b) Slow rising pulse

- I is the intensity of the current; on the machine this is controlled by the intensity control to each pair of electrodes.
- D is the duration of the pulse or pulse width; this is pre-set on some machines but others have a pulse width control. A pulse width of under 100 μs is not effective and the best results are obtained with pulse widths of between 200 and 300 μs.
- Some machines produce pulses of different shapes.
- The shape of the pulse is known as the wave form (see Figure 5.10).

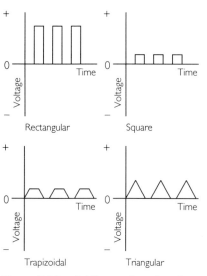

Figure 5.10   *Different shaped pulses*

Figure 5.11   *Pulses of different frequency*

- It is the rate of rise of each pulse that determines the response in the muscle. A pulse which rises sharply produces the best response in innervated muscle and the rectangular pulse is generally used in beauty therapy units.

- A single, adequate pulse will produce a twitch in the muscle. The muscle contracts as the current rises and the contraction diminishes as the current falls; the muscle relaxes completely when the current stops.

- If a number of pulses are applied to the muscle, the type of contraction produced will depend on the interval between the pulses.

- If the interval between pulses is long enough for the muscle to relax, then a series of twitches will be produced in the muscle giving a tremulous contraction.

- If the pulses follow each other in rapid succession, the muscle has no time to relax and a smooth contraction is produced. A smooth contraction of a muscle is known as a *tetanic* contraction.

- The number of pulses produced every second is known as the frequency and is measured in Hz.

These pulses with a long interval in between allow the muscle to relax, thus producing a series of twitches

These pulses with short intervals in between do not allow the muscle to relax, thus producing a smooth fused contraction

FREQUENCY

- The frequency of the pulses is an important consideration because the different fibres within a muscle will respond in a different way to various frequencies.

- Below 20 Hz (ie pulses per second) only the slow fibres will be showing smooth, fused tetanic contractions; the faster fibres will be showing unfused contractions.

- As the frequency is increased to 40 Hz, the majority of fibres will be showing fused tetanic contractions, although some fast fibres may require higher frequencies to produce maximum force.

- At 60 Hz, the majority of fast fibres will be showing smooth, fused tetanic contractions and the whole muscle will contract smoothly. This can be represented diagramatically as follows:

Figure 5.12 *Muscle contraction at different frequency*

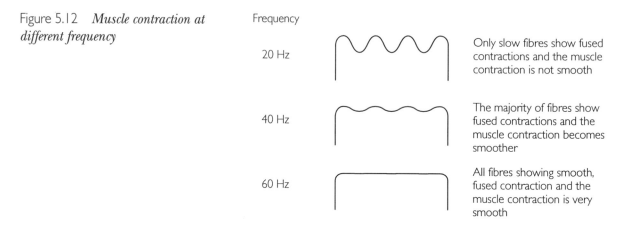

- In most human muscle, maximal force is developed in the frequency range of 40–80 Hz, and there is nothing to be gained by using higher frequencies. The highest frequency recorded during normal transmission is around 100 Hz.

CONTRACTION TIME

C is the contraction time
R is the relaxation time

Figure 5.13 *Trains or envelopes of pulses*

- The pulses are grouped together in 'trains' or 'envelopes', with a rest period in between. When the current flows, the muscle contracts; when the current stops, the muscle relaxes.
- On most machines, the contraction and relaxation period can be varied.
- In order to improve client comfort, the pulse envelope is surged so that the strength of the pulses rise gradually to peak intensity.
- The current may then stop suddenly on some units, or decrease gradually on others.

Figure 5.14 *Surged envelopes*

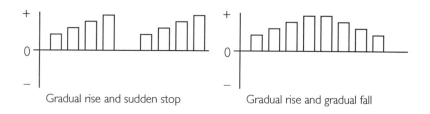

- The rate of rise of the current is known as the ramp time.

PHASIC SELECTION

Monophasic–all the pulses are in one direction

Biphasic–alternate pulses are reversed

Figure 5.15 *Monophasic and Biphasic pulses*

- Many units have a phasic control and offer a choice of monophasic or biphasic current.
- With monophasic current, the current flows mainly in one direction, ie electrons flow from the negative electrode (cathode) to the positive electrode (anode) without variation. Consequently, the negative electrode will produce the stronger contraction. This is an important consideration when using duplicate or split padding (see page 80). The negative electrode (cathode) should always be placed on the weaker muscle or weaker side and should also be used as the mushroom electrode for the stimulation of individual muscles, the indifferent anode being placed elsewhere.
- With biphasic current, each alternate pulse is reversed so that with the first pulse electron flow is from cathode to anode but the second pulse flow is reversed. In this way polarity is cancelled out and even strength contractions are produced under each pad.

TYPES OF ELECTRODES

Figure 5.16

The current is conducted from the machine to the client by means of leads and electrodes. These electrodes come in various forms:

1 *Rubber pads.* These are the most common form of electrode. They are made of rubber impregnated with a good conductor, such as graphite. They come in various sizes and may be round or square. Only one side is conductive, the other side is rubber insulated.
2 *Metal plates.* These are no longer used with modern equipment. They are made of tin, cut to the required size and attached to the lead with a clip. They were placed on top of 16 layers of lint.
3 *Mushroom or disc electrodes.* These are metal discs on the end of wooden handles. The discs are covered with 16 layers of lint. They are useful for individual stimulation of small muscles.
4 *Facial electrode.* This has both electrodes, the anode and cathode, set into an insulating holder. It is used to stimulate facial muscles.
5 *Facial mask electrode.* This has many electrodes fitted into the mask. It covers the face and stimulates the muscles simultaneously.
6 *Roller electrodes.* These are small metal cylinders covered with lint. They are used for labile treatments on large sheets of muscle, such as the back muscles. The roller is moved slowly over the back stimulating the muscles as it passes over the motor points.

The placement of pads (electrodes)

The correct placement of pads is very important and will affect the outcome of the treatment. In order to pad effectively, the therapist must understand the methods of padding and must know the position of the motor points of the superficial muscles. A pad placed anywhere on the muscle will initiate a response, but may well be uncomfortable. The most effective and comfortable contraction is obtained if a muscle is stimulated at the motor point, ie where the nerve enters the muscle belly (see page 73). Motor point padding should always be used if possible, as it allows very precise targeting of muscles and enables suitable intensities to be selected for individual muscles. Stimulation here is more effective at lower intensities and is therefore more comfortable for the client. Bilateral padding is usually used in beauty therapy as improvement is required on both sides of the body. Various names are given to varieties of padding.

LONGITUDINAL PADDING

In the past, this method used the pads near the origin and insertion of the muscle. However, as muscle function may be impaired by padding off the motor points, longitudinal padding must now mean padding on the upper and lower motor points of a muscle. This is only possible on long muscles with more than one motor point. This is an excellent method of motor point padding as all the current is applied to one muscle and the intensity is controlled to gain maximum contraction of the muscle. Also as the current from one pair of pads is applied to one muscle, a lower intensity will produce the desired contraction, which will be more comfortable for the client. This would always be the method of choice for muscles with two motor points. The next pair of pads is applied to the same muscle on the other side of the body. Muscles which may be padded longitudinally include: *rectus abdominis, rectus femoris, gracilis, trapezius, triceps.*

DUPLICATE PADDING

A pair of pads is placed on the motor points of two adjacent muscles; the next pair is placed on the same two muscles on the other side of the body. This method has the disadvantage that the intensity cannot be controlled to individual muscles, and muscles may require different intensities if one is weaker than another. The use of monophasic pulses will help if the cathode is placed on the weaker muscle. As the current is divided, a higher intensity may be required to produce the desired contraction and will be less comfortable for the client. When using duplicate motor point padding, always try to pad muscles with the same or similar action.

Muscles which are suitable for duplicate padding include: *gluteus medius* and *tensor fasciae latae* (abductors); *adductor longus* and *gracilis* (adductors); *external oblique* and *rectus abdominis* (abdominals).

SPLIT PADDING

One pair of pads is split and placed on the motor point of the same muscle, but on opposite sides of the body. Again the current is divided between two muscles, which prevents individual control. If one side of the body is weaker than the other, monophasic pulses should be used and the cathode placed on the weaker muscle. If muscles are of equal strength, biphasic pulses should be used. This is a useful method for using up the last pair of pads. Muscles suitable for split padding include: right and left *pectorals*; right and left *triceps*; right and left *gluteus maximus*.

FACTORS TO BE BORNE IN MIND WHEN PADDING

1 Always pad on motor points if possible.
2 Use longitudinal padding if a muscle has more than one motor point. The intensity can be selected to obtain maximum contraction of that muscle.
3 For optimum contraction, place a muscle in its relaxed mid range position.
4 The brain does not register individual muscle movement, but rather patterns of movement. During normal body movement, antagonistic muscles do not contract together. When the prime mover contracts, the antagonist relaxes. Therefore, when simulating movement, the padding of opposite muscles should be avoided. In practice it is not always possible to adhere rigidly to this rule, and providing there is no movement at the joint, opposing muscles are sometimes padded, eg the adductors and abductors of the hip joint.

   Some units are designed to stimulate antagonistic muscles alternately, this would seem a good idea.

   When using duplicate padding, do not use one pair on antagonistic muscles as one is likely to be weaker than the other and the intensity to each group cannot be individually controlled.
5 Consider the phase control when padding. With biphasic current the contractions are even under both pads. With monophasic current the cathode is stronger and should

therefore be used where one muscle of a pair may be weaker than the other (very useful for duplicate and split padding).

Methods of padding should be selected and adapted to suit the needs of individual clients. Having decided on padding methods, other factors should be considered which will influence the response.

1 Thoroughly cleansing the skin to remove sebum and dirt (wash with warm soapy water or use cologne).
2 Pre-heating the muscles with some form of heat treatment will increase the response, eg infrared, sauna, or steam bath (which is particularly effective as it also moistens the skin).
3 Ensuring the accurate positioning of electrodes/pads on the motor points.
4 Selecting appropriate control settings.

Remember that fat impedes the flow of current, and the treatment will be ineffective if the muscles are covered by a deep layer of fat. Muscle stimulation is also ineffective on deep muscles. Padding should be selected for superficial muscles only.

Superficial body and facial motor points

Figure 5.17   *Motor points of the facial muscles*

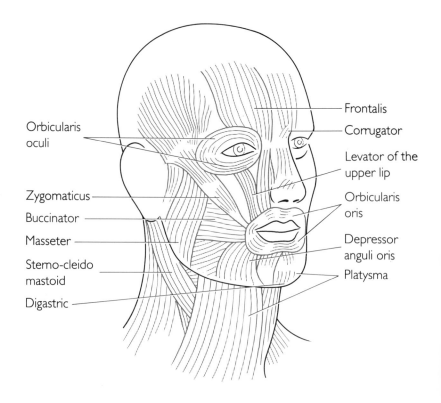

Figure 5.18   *Skeletal muscles and motor points (anterior)*

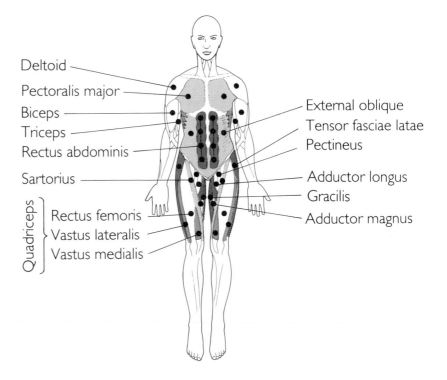

Deltoid

Pectoralis major

Biceps

Triceps

Rectus abdominis

Sartorius

Quadriceps {
Rectus femoris

Vastus lateralis

Vastus medialis
}

External oblique

Tensor fasciae latae

Pectineus

Adductor longus

Gracilis

Adductor magnus

Figure 5.19   *Skeletal muscles and motor points (posterior)*

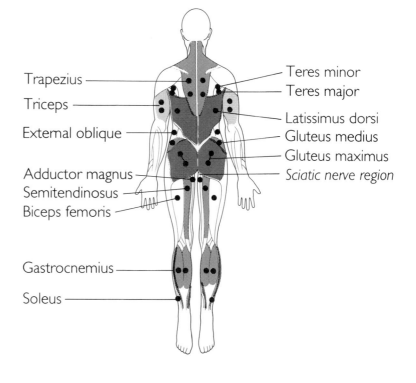

Trapezius

Triceps

External oblique

Adductor magnus

Semitendinosus

Biceps femoris

Gastrocnemius

Soleus

Teres minor

Teres major

Latissimus dorsi

Gluteus medius

Gluteus maximus

Sciatic nerve region

Stimulation of facial muscles

The machines for facial stimulation are very simple units with an on/off switch and an intensity control to one pair of electrodes; some have a surge control. Some of the large body machines include a special terminal for facial stimulation.

Figure 5.20 *Electrical muscle stimulator showing combined facial electrode*

METHODS OF APPLICATION

1 *Disc electrode.* This electrode is used on the motor point of the muscle and is known as the active electrode; a plate electrode, which is placed behind the shoulder or strapped to the arms, is known as the inactive electrode. Specific muscles are stimulated in turn six to eight contractions per muscle. The procedure is repeated three times.

2 *Facial electrode.* Here a plastic or rubber holder contains both the active and the inactive electrode. It is placed over a group of muscles or a branch of the facial nerve, and these are stimulated six to eight times and repeated three times. This method does not produce specific movement of individual muscles, but the simultaneous contractions of many muscles.

3 *Facial mask.* Here there are electrodes within a mask which is placed over the face. The muscles are stimulated simultaneously. Treatment lasts for 10 minutes. Some clients find this mask claustrophobic.

USES

1 Ageing skin – wrinkled with poor elasticity.
2 Loss of firm contours due to muscle weakness.
3 As a preventative measure to delay the effects of ageing and promote cellular function.
4 Slight puffiness around the eyes.

EFFECTS

1 It improves muscle tone and the general condition of the muscle. This results in improvement of the contours of the face.
2 The pumping action increases the supply of blood to the skin and muscle, thus bringing nutrients and oxygen to the body part and removing waste products. This results in improved condition of skin and muscle.
3 Vasodilation giving erythema.
4 The contraction and relaxation of muscles aids the removal of fluid from the area; it relieves swelling.
5 It irritates sensory nerve endings.

CONTRA-INDICATIONS

1 Highly strung or nervous client.
2 Hypersensitive skins (the current will irritate the skin further).
3 Highly vascular complexions.
4 High blood pressure.
5 Sinus congestion.
6 Headaches or migraine.
7 Many skin abrasions.
8 Over superficial bony areas.
9 Large number of fillings or bridgework.
10 Epileptic or diabetic client.

PRECAUTIONS

1 Check that all jewellery has been removed.
2 Check for contra-indications.
3 Cleanse the skin.
4 Test the machine.
5 If there is a surge control, select the correct length of surge to suit the client (longer surge for poor muscle tone).
6 Ensure that the intensity controls are at zero.
7 Dampen pads with saline and ensure that they remain moist throughout the treatment.
8 Turn up during surge only when the light is on.
9 Always turn off before moving the electrode (*Note:* do not move the electrode with the intensity turned up).
10 Do not over treat – six to eight contractions per muscle are required and repeated three times.

TREATMENT TECHNIQUE

Figure 5.21   *Stimulation of facial motor points with disc electrode*

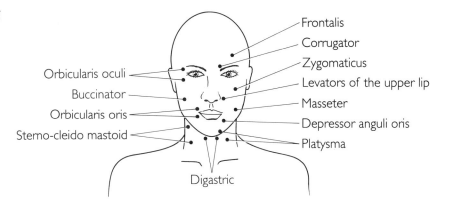

PREPARATION OF THE CLIENT

1 Place the client in a well supported comfortable position.
2 Check that all jewellery has been removed.
3 Cleanse the face thoroughly – tone the skin to remove all grease as this is a barrier to the current.
4 Check for contra-indications, particularly for any abrasions, and cover these with petroleum jelly or plaster.
5 Explain the treatment to the client, ie a prickling sensation giving way to contraction. Ask her to report any discomfort.

PROCEDURE

1 Prepare the machine, place it on a stable base and check that the plugs and leads are secure.
2 Check that the intensity controls are at zero.
3 Collect commodities: hot water or saline solution and cotton wool.
4 Prepare the electrodes; select the cathode as the active disc electrode (cover them with 16 layers of lint if necessary).
5 Moisten the electrode cover.
6 Check the current on yourself (hold both electrodes in one hand).
7 Turn the dials back to zero.
8 If using a single disc electrode, strap the indifferent electrode behind the shoulder.
9 Place the electrode in position on the face.
10 Tell the client that the machine is being switched on.
11 Turn up the intensity control slowly until a prickling sensation is felt; continue increasing the intensity until a contraction is obtained.

12 After six to eight contractions, turn the intensity down to zero.

13 Move the electrode to the next muscle and repeat the procedure. Repeat three times.

14 If using a mask electrode, treat the client for 10–15 minutes.

15 When the treatment is complete, turn the intensity to zero, remove the electrode and switch the machine off.

16 Wipe toner over the treated area.

17 Advise on facial exercises for home care.

18 Remove and dispose of lint cover, wipe the electrode with disinfectant wipe.

19 Treatment time 10–15 minutes.

Note:

1 Talk to the client and reassure her during the treatment.

2 Always turn up the intensity during the surge period.

3 Do not over treat as this will cause muscle fatigue.

4 The therapist should be able to see the machine and the client at all times, and be in easy reach of controls.

REASONS FOR POOR CONTRACTIONS

1 The intensity is too low (not enough current to initiate a contraction).

2 The pads are too dry or dirty (wet, clean pads are better conductors of current; dirty pads offer resistance).

3 Grease on the skin (grease is a barrier to the current).

4 Incorrect positioning of the pads or mask (padding accurately over the motor point gives the best contraction, as this is the point of maximum excitability).

5 Poor contact between the skin and the electrode (gaps offer resistance to current).

6 Poor contact or loose terminals (the current will not flow if the circuit is broken).

Figure 5.22   *Body treatment*

Stimulation of superficial body muscles

The machines for body muscle stimulation are very complex and they have multiple outlets. The controls vary in number and in terminology. The therapist must familiarise herself with the machines she is using in order to select the settings to suit the client.

MACHINE CONTROLS

1 *On/off switch.* This switches the current on and off; there is usually a light which comes on to show that the current is flowing.

2 *Surge control/surge envelope/contraction time/stimulation period.* This controls the length of time the current is flowing, ie the length of the surge envelope or train; it controls the length of time the muscle contracts. While the current flows, the muscle contracts; when the current stops, the muscle relaxes. The surge length should be long enough to produce a good contraction. Muscles with poor tone or with a thick layer of covering fat require a longer surge. The surge control usually varies from $\frac{1}{2}$ second to $2\frac{1}{2}$ seconds.

Figure 5.23   *Electronic surges of different length*

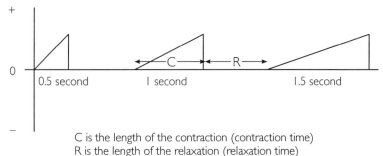

C is the length of the contraction (contraction time)
R is the length of the relaxation (relaxation time)

3 *Relaxation control/interval or rest period.* This controls the length of the rest period between the contractions. The rest period should be equal to, or slightly longer than, the surge period; this allows the muscle to relax fully, preventing muscle fatigue and build up of lactic acid which would cause pain. It should not be too long as this is a waste of time. Many modern machines have an inbuilt automatic optimum relaxation time.

4 *Ramp-time.* This controls the rate of rise of the current; individual pulses are inhibited gradually to give build up to peak flow. Sharp rises give the best response. The rate must not be too slow as the muscle will accommodate.

5 *Frequency control/pulses per second/Hz.* This controls the number of pulses per second. The importance of frequency is discussed fully on page 77. Frequency determines the strength of contraction at the motor unit. Different fibre types will respond differently to different frequencies (see page 74). Up to 20 Hz, only the slow fibres will be showing smooth, fused tetanic contraction. At 40 Hz, the majority of fibres will be showing fused tetanic contractions, although some fast fibres may require a higher frequency. Therefore, by selecting a frequency of 40 to 60 Hz, most fibres in the muscle will be contracting smoothly.

The frequency within this range can be selected to provide the most comfortable smooth contraction for the client. If there is a tremor in the muscle, a higher frequency is needed. There is nothing to be gained by selecting frequencies over 80 Hz as near maximal force is developed in human muscle with frequencies between 40 and 80 Hz. Some machines offer timed sequences beginning with lower frequencies moving through middle into higher frequencies.

6 *Phase control.* This offers biphasic or monophasic pulses.
   (a) Monophasic/uniphasic/single pulses. The current flows mainly in one direction; therefore, the polarity of the pads remains the same for each contraction. One will be $(-)$, the cathode, and the other $(+)$, the anode. Leads usually indicate this by one having a groove or being rounded – check with the manufacturer's instructions to establish which is which. As the cathode produces the greatest response, it should always be placed on the weaker muscle. This is useful for split and duplicate motor point padding if one muscle is weaker than another. If muscles are of equal power, and for longitudinal padding, biphasic pulses may be used.
   (b) Biphasic/dual pulses. The current behaves like AC as alternate pulses are reversed; it therefore eliminates polarity. It provides an even current under both pads.

7 *Mode control/programme control.* This controls the rhythms of the contraction and relaxation times.
   (a) Constant. The rhythm of the programme remains the same once selected. The length of surge and interval remain the same throughout treatment.
   (b) Variable/rhythmic/active. The rhythm of the surge and interval vary throughout the treatment. This has the advantage of preventing the client anticipating the contraction and resisting it (useful with tense, nervous clients). In many modern machines, a selection of variable contraction times will give the muscles thorough non-repetitious exercise.

8 *Pulse width.* This alters the width of each pulse; when the pulse width is increased, it has a similar effect to increasing the intensity control. This is because additional current is provided as the pulse is on for a longer period. Pulse widths under 100 µs are not effective; over 300 µs can be uncomfortable. A medium width of between 200 and 300 µs produces a good contraction. Select 150–200 µs at the commencement of treatment, and if the client cannot tolerate an increase in intensity due to discomfort, increase the pulse width, which may produce a better contraction.

9 *Maximum and minimum gain/master output.* This control increases the current to all the outlets being used – to increase the intensity when the client has got used to sensation. This control can be at zero at commencement of treatment, or it can be set midway so that the intensity can be increased or decreased during treatment.

10 *Intensity controls (output controls) and pulse amplitude.* These control the current flowing through each pair of pads. Most machines have an intensity control for one pair of pads, however, there are machines where two pairs of pads share the same intensity control.

As the intensity control is turned up, the amount of current flowing through the pad increases. When selecting intensity, 'a good visible contraction within the tolerance of the client' is the best guide. Avoid turning the intensity too high thinking that a stronger contraction is always better. Muscle fibres obey the 'all or none law', ie once the stimulus is great enough to produce a contraction, there will be no increase in response by turning up the intensity. However, as the intensity of the current is increased, the strength of contraction is seen to increase. This is because more motor units are stimulated. Some machines have numbers around the intensity control which serve as a rough guide. The intensity control will be turned up to obtain optimum maximum contraction with minimum discomfort.

FACTORS GOVERNING THE STRENGTH OF THE CONTRACTIONS

Many factors influence the strength of contractions. Output controls regulate the amount of current flowing to the tissues, but are little guide to the amount of contraction. The strength of contraction varies and depends on many factors:

1 The size of the muscle and the selection of appropriate padding.
2 The number of motor units activated.
3 The depth of the muscle – EMS is effective on superficial muscle only.
4 The amount of covering fat – fat is an insulator; therefore, current will not pass through very fatty areas.
5 The condition of the muscle – well-toned muscles respond to lower intensity of current.
6 The rate of rise of the current – a sharp rise produces a contraction, a slow rise allows for accommodation of the muscle fibres.
7 Moist skin offers less resistance to the current.
8 Warm muscles contract more readily.
9 Firm, even padding giving good surface contact will ensure maximum effect.

Uses

1 Figure reshaping, particularly when used in conjunction with active exercise.
2 To re-educate muscles with poor tone due to prolonged disuse, eg adductors and triceps.
3 To restore muscle tone of abdominals after pregnancy.
4 To firm the pectoral muscles, which may correct breast sag.
5 To firm body contours and maintain an attractive figure, while losing body weight through dieting.

Physiological effects

1 The stimulation of motor nerves resulting in muscle contraction. The selection of an appropriate frequency will produce contraction of most fibres of a muscle. (This differs from active movement when only a percentage of fibres contract; it therefore improves muscle tone.)
2 It improves the circulation due to the pumping action of the contracting muscles. This increases the nutrients and oxygen brought to the body part and speeds up the removal of waste products.
3 It increases the metabolic rate, which improves the condition of the muscle.
4 It stimulates the sensory nerve, giving the prickling sensation.
5 It produces vasodilation and erythema under the pads.

Contra-indications

1 Muscle injury or spasm.
2 Broken bones.
3 Extensive cuts and bruises (small cuts may be insulated with petroleum jelly).
4 Skin disorders and diseases.
5 Recent scar tissue.
6 Metal pins and plates (superficial).
7 Pacemakers.
8 Heart conditions.
9 High or low blood pressure.
10 Thrombosis.
11 Phlebitis.
12 Do not pad heavily in the chest region near the heart.

Dangers

● There are no specific dangers to EMS. Discomfort can be caused if the intensity is too high, if the pads are in the wrong position, ie not on motor points, over bony points or over any open abrasions that are not insulated.

- Muscle fatigue can be produced if the intensity is too high, the rest interval is too short or the treatment is prolonged.
- Turn on the machine during surge so that the client can feel the intensity increasing and let you know if it is too high.
- Turn the machine off during the rest period.
- Heavy padding of the chest region should be avoided as stimuli may interfere with heart rhythm.

PRECAUTIONS

1 When the intensity is turned up, *never* move the pads, press pads down or push the terminals in.
2 Check for contra-indications.
3 Test the machine.
4 Select appropriate points on all controls.
5 Ensure the intensity controls are at zero.
6 Check the pads and wet them with saline or water.
7 Strap the pads securely.
8 Check the outlets before switching the machine on.
9 Turn *up* during the *surge* only.
10 Avoid heavy padding of chest region, pad anterior or posterior but not both.

TREATMENT TECHNIQUE

PREPARATION OF THE CLIENT

1 Position the client in a comfortable, well-supported position.
2 Remove jewellery.
3 Check for contra-indications.
4 Pre-heat the body using steam, sauna, infrared/radiant heat or shower – this improves muscle action and moistens the skin, thus lowering its resistance.
5 Explain the treatment to the client, eg a prickling sensation followed by contraction; reassure the patient and encourage her to relax.

PROCEDURE

1 Place the machine on a suitable stable base and check that the plugs and leads are secure.
2 Check that the intensity controls are at zero.
3 Collect all commodities, hot water or saline solution, cotton

wool, talc, cologne and a selection of straps of varying lengths.

4 Check the machine on yourself.

5 Check skin for cuts, abrasions and insulate them with petroleum jelly or cover with plaster. If the client has not taken a shower clean the skin by washing or wiping with cologne or surgical spirit.

6 Select a suitable padding layout and make a note of it on a record card.

7 Secure the straps around the body.

8 Moisten the surfaces of the pads evenly and place them accurately over the identified motor points; ensure a firm even contact.

9 Select the appropriate controls, frequency, mode, etc.

10 Check that the intensity controls are at zero.

11 Switch the machine on and turn each intensity control up slowly until a good visible contraction is obtained.

12 Cover the client and keep her warm.

13 As the client grows accustomed to the sensation, and as pads dry out slightly, the intensity may be increased after a few minutes.

14 The treatment should end after 30–40 minutes. Switch off.

15 Turn all dials to zero.

16 Remove the pads in reverse order to avoid tangling.

17 Dry and talc treated area.

18 Clean the pads with warm water and detergent.

19 The treatment can be carried out two to three times per week for six to eight weeks as required.

20 The client should be taught exercises to carry out at home to increase the effectiveness of the treatment.

REASONS FOR POOR CONTRACTIONS

1 The intensity is too low.

2 The pads are too dry or dirty.

3 There is grease on the skin.

4 Treating over a depth of fat.

5 Incorrect positioning of pads (off motor points or near tendons).

6 Poor contact between the pads and skin.

7 Poor contact at leads and loose terminals.

PATTERNS OF PADDING FOR USE ON THE BODY

In order to pad accurately, therapists must understand the three methods of padding and the position of the motor points of the superficial body muscles. Padding should then be selected to suit the client. Some suggestions are shown in figure 5.24.

Therapists need to remember that the long or large abdomen

Figure 5.24 *Suggested methods for body padding*

Longitudinal padding for a tall client with a long or large abdomen.
Pads 1 and 2 on the first and third motor points of Rectus Abdominis. Pads 3 and 4 on the second and fourth motor points of Rectus Abdominis. Pads 5 and 6 on the External Oblique and pads 7 and 8 on Gracilis. Pads 9 and 10 use duplicate padding on Tensor Fasciae Latae, and Gluteus Medius

Padding for a short client with small abdomen.
Pads 1 and 2 longitudinal on Rectus Abdominis. Pads 3 and 4 duplicate on External Oblique and Rectus Abdominis. Pads 5 and 6 duplicate on Adductor longus and Gracilis. Pads 7 and 8 duplicate on Tensor Fasciae Latae and Gluteus Medius. Pads 9 and 10 could be placed longitudinally on Gluteus Maximus

Padding for chest abdominals and hips and buttocks.
1 and 2 longitudinal Pectoralis Major. 3 and 4 longitudinal Rectus Abdominis. 5 and 6 duplicate Rectus Abdominis and External Oblique. 7 and 8 duplicate Tensor Fasciae Latae and Gluteus Medius and 9 and 10 longitudinal Gluteus Maximus

Padding for buttocks and thighs using duplicate padding throughout. 1 and 2 Sartorius & Rectus Femoris. 3 and 4 Tensor Fasciae Latae and Vastus Lateralis. 5 and 6 on Gracilis and Vastus Medialis. 7 and 8 on Gluteus Maximus and Gluteus Medius and 9 and 10 on Gluteus Maximus and Biceps Femoris

Padding to strengthen the back. Pads 1 and 2 longitudinal on Trapezius. Pads 3 and 4 longitudinal on Latissimus Dorsi. Pad 5 is split on Right and Left Triceps. Pads 6 and 7 duplicate on Gluteus Medius and Tensor Fascia Lata. Pads 8 and 9 longitudinal on Gluteus Maximus. Pad 10 Split on Gracilis requires more pads than the small abdomen so use the four motor points of Rectus abdominis and pad External oblique longitudinally. The Internal oblique and Transverus Abdominis are too deep for stimulation. For the abductor muscles, Tensor Fasciae Latae, Gluteus Medius and the deep Minimus which give shape to the thigh, insert high up on the thigh. Gluteus Medius & the deep Minimus both insert into the greater trochanter of the femur, but Tensor Fasciae Latae inserts into the lateral fascia of the thigh. Therefore padding on the top and bottom of the outside of the thigh will not target these muscles. This method of padding will target Tensor Fasciae Latae and Vastus Lateralis.

In the past beauty therapists have avoided padding the Quadriceps group as their strength is maintained through constant use. However, there is now a growing desire among some members of the general public for athletic looking legs and quadriceps can be padded to achieve this aim. The quadriceps muscles could be padded as follows: Rectus femoris may be duplicated with Sartorius, Vastus medialis may be duplicated with Gracilis, Vastus lateralis may be duplicated with Tensor fasciae latae. Vastus intermedius is too deep for stimulation.

Triceps may be padded longitudinally or split. This will improve the tone at the posterior aspect of the upper arm. Biceps rarely needs improvement in tone as it is in constant use. Do not stimulate biceps and triceps together as contraction of these muscles will move the elbow joint.

Placing the client in a low half-lying position will achieve better abdominal contractions as the muscles are relaxed and will contract in mid range.

SUMMARY

- Electrical impulses produced by machines will stimulate motor nerves resulting in the contraction of muscles supplied by those nerves.
- Muscles are composed of bundles of muscle fibres.
- Motor nerves (or neurones) transmit impulses from the brain and spinal cord to the muscle fibres.
- The *motor end plate* is the modification of the muscle fibre at the point where the nerve terminal comes close to it. The synapse between the end of the nerve and the muscle fibre it supplies is known as the *neuro-muscular junction.*
- The *motor point* is the point where the motor nerve enters the belly of the muscle; after entering the muscle it divides into many branches. Each branch supplies a single muscle fibre.
- The *motor unit* includes the anterior horn cell, its axon, axon branches and all the muscle fibres supplied by that axon.

- One motor unit will supply hundreds of muscle fibres, therefore, many motor units are required to supply a whole muscle.

- Each muscle is made up of different types of muscle fibres, ie slow oxidative fibres, fast oxidative glycolytic fibres and fast glycolytic fibres.

- These fibres respond in different ways to different rates of frequencies of impulses: slow fibres contract smoothly, ie tetanically, to low frequencies up to 20 Hz; fast fibres contract smoothly, ie tetanically, to higher frequencies up to 80 Hz.

- Smooth, tetanic muscle contraction is obtained at frequencies of between 40–80 Hz.

ELECTRICAL STIMULATION

- Pulses must be of sufficient duration and intensity to produce a contraction (high frequency currents have pulses of short duration and will not stimulate motor nerves).

- A sharply rising pulse produces the best contraction; slow rising pulses allow the muscle to accommodate. Pulses are grouped together in trains or envelopes with rest periods in between.

- When the current flows, the muscles contract; when the current stops, the muscles relax.

- Pulses are surged so that each pulse increases in intensity to peak value and then decreases. The rate of rise of the current is known as the ramp time. The frequency of the current is the number of pulses per second. Different muscle fibres respond differently to different frequencies. Only slow fibres will contract smoothly/tetanically to frequencies under 20 Hz, the fast fibres require frequencies of around 60 to 80 Hz to produce smooth tetanic contractions.

- Frequencies in the range 40–80 Hz will produce good tetanic contractions when using EMS. A few minutes at the lower range of 20 Hz, moving into middle range 40–60 Hz and then to 80 Hz and back to middle gives a thorough treatment.

- The intensity selected should produce 'a good visible contraction' within the tolerance of the client.

PHASIC CONTROLS

- Monophasic selection means that one pad is slightly stronger than the other; the cathode is stronger than the anode. This may be used for duplicate or split padding if one muscle is weaker than the other when the cathode would be used on the weaker muscle.

- Biphasic selection means that alternate pulses are reversed, which eliminates polarity; the current is even under both pads.

This may be used with longitudinal padding or with other methods if the muscles are of equal strength.

- The pulse width selected is between 200 and 300 μs.
- Always use motor point padding.
- There are three methods used on the body:

1 Longitudinal: a pair of pads are on one muscle, one on the upper motor point, the other on the lower motor point. Repeat this on the other side of the body.
2 Duplicate: a pair of pads are on two adjacent muscles, one on the motor point of one muscle, the other on the motor point of the other muscle. Repeat this on the other side of the body.
3 Split padding: a pair of pads are on the same muscle, but on opposite sides of the body, one on the motor point of the right muscle, the other on the motor point of the left muscle.

- There are two methods commonly used on the face:

1 Facial disc electrode: a disc is used as the active electrode and is used over the motor point of individual muscles. The inactive electrode is strapped on to the arm or behind the shoulder.
2 Facial inactive and active combined electrode: this contains both electrodes, and is placed over the branches of the facial nerve to stimulate many muscles simultaneously.

QUESTIONS

1 Describe the composition of skeletal muscle.
2 List the parts of the nervous system.
3 Define the following:
   (a) motor point,
   (b) neuro-muscular junction,
   (c) motor end plate,
   (d) motor unit.
4 List three types of muscle fibres and give the transmission frequencies to produce smooth contractions of each fibre type.
5 Why should the electrodes/pads be placed on the motor point of a muscle?
6 Give three uses for electrical muscle stimulation of the face.
7 Explain three methods used for padding superficial body muscles.
8 Explain the difference in muscle response when using a disc electrode or a combined facial electrode when stimulating facial muscles.
9 Explain the purpose of the following controls found on machines:

   (a) intensity control,
   (b) surge length,
   (c) relaxation length,
   (d) phasic control,
   (e) pulse width,
   (f) maximum/minimum gain or master control,
   (g) rhythm control.
10 The intensity of current is one factor that governs the strength of contractions; list six other factors which determine the strength of contractions.
11 List six contra-indications to each of the following:
   (a) stimulation of facial muscles,
   (b) stimulation of body muscles.
12 Give three uses for electrical muscle stimulation of body muscles.
13 Give the dangers to electrical stimulation of body muscles.
14 Describe four factors which may result in poor contractions.

CHAPTER 6   *Galvanic treatment*

Figure 6.1   *Combined facial and body galvanic unit*

OBJECTIVES

After you have studied this chapter you will be able to:

1 Identify a galvanic unit, its terminals and electrodes.
2 List the treatments which use the galvanic current.
3 Describe the type of current used in galvanic treatments.
4 Briefly explain the chemical electrolysis of sodium chloride solution (salt or saline solution).
5 Briefly describe the effects of galvanic treatment to the body using the pads soaked in salt solution.
6 Explain the uses of disincrustation treatment.
7 Carry out disincrustation treatment paying due consideration to maximum efficiency, comfort, safety and hygiene.
8 Explain the uses of iontophoresis treatment.
9 Carry out iontophoresis treatment paying due consideration to maximum efficiency, comfort, safety and hygiene.
10 Explain the uses of body galvanism.
11 Explain the dangers of galvanic application to the body.
12 List the precautions to be taken during galvanic application to the body.
13 Treat the client with body galvanism paying due consideration to maximum efficiency, comfort, safety and hygiene.

Figure 6.1 is a photograph of a galvanic machine or unit. This is one of the larger models and is used for both facial and body work. Galvanic treatments use a low voltage direct (constant) current, sometimes called a galvanic current. This current flows in one direction only and has polarity. One electrode is negatively charged (called the *cathode*), while the other is positively charged (called the *anode*). Galvanic treatments may be used on the face or body and are given specific names:

1 Disincrustation – a facial treatment. This is a deep cleansing treatment; the effects at the cathode are used to remove the build up of sebum and keratinised cells and to soften the skin of the face.
2 Iontophoresis or ion repulsion – facial and body treatment. This treatment uses specially manufactured products which are repelled into the skin by appropriate electrodes. It is suitable for many skin types as a variety of products are available to suit different skin conditions. For body treatments, anti-cellulite products are used to soften and aid the dispersal of hard fat (cellulite).
3 Body galvanism – body treatment. This treatment uses the softening effect under the cathode when using a sodium chloride (salt solution) under the electrode, to treat areas of cellulite.

4 Epilation or hair removal – This treatment is based on the principle of electrolysis but is not covered in this book.

The effects produced by these treatments are dependent on:

1 The chemistry of electrolysis.
2 The laws of physics which state that like charges repel and opposite charges attract.

The first part of this chapter explains these principles, and it is advantageous for all therapists to study and understand them before commencing treatments. This knowledge will enable the therapist to select the most appropriate and effective treatment to suit the needs of the client. It will also enable her to fully explain the treatment to the client.

Revision

Read the sections on elements (see page 3), compounds (see page 3), atoms (see page 4), ions (see page 6) and electrolytes (page 8).

Electrolysis of sodium chloride solution

A solution containing salt and water is an electrolyte. In solution, the sodium chloride will ionise and the water will ionise slightly.

Sodium chloride will ionise giving sodium (+) ions and chloride (−) ions

$$NaCl \rightarrow Na^+ \text{ and } Cl^-$$

Water will ionise giving hydrogen (+) ions and hydroxyl (−) ions

$$H_2O \rightarrow H^+ \text{ and } OH^-$$

These ions move freely in the solution; when a direct current is applied to the solution by means of two electrodes, the current will flow through the electrolyte. The electrodes will be charged depending on their connections to the battery or machine. One will be negatively charged, the *cathode*. The other will be positively charged, the *anode*. When the current is switched on, the ions will move away from or towards the electrodes. This occurs because:

1 Like charges repel.
2 Opposite charges attract.

Therefore, the cations (+) will move towards the cathode (−) and the anions (−) will move towards the anode (+).

Figure 6.2 *Electrolysis of sodium chloride solution*

When the ions reach the electrode with the opposite charge, some are discharged and certain chemical reactions take place. The following reactions are used in galvanic treatments.

- At the cathode ($-$) the sodium ion (Na^+) reacts with the hydroxyl ion (OH^-) in the water producing the alkali sodium hydroxide ($NaOH$) and hydrogen (H_2) gas.
- At the anode ($+$) the chloride ion (Cl^-) reacts with the hydrogen ions (H^+) in the water producing hydrochloric acid (HCl) and Oxygen (O_2) gas.

The above can be represented as equations (numbers are used to balance the equation).

Sodium + water $\longrightarrow$ sodium hydroxide + hydrogen
$2Na + 2H_2O \longrightarrow 2NaOH + H_2$

Chlorine + water $\longrightarrow$ hydrochloric acid + oxygen
$2Cl_2 + 2H_2O \longrightarrow 4HCl + O_2$

The formation of the alkali sodium hydroxide at the cathode is used in facial disincrustation and body galvanism. A current applied to the body by means of two electrodes will be carried through the tissues. This happens because tissue fluid contains a high percentage of salts and is an electrolyte. A pad of lint or foam soaked in salt solution and placed under the cathode and moved over or strapped to the skin will result in the production of sodium hydroxide under the pad. This has a softening effect on the tissues. At the same time, hydrochloric acid will be produced under the anode. This hardens the tissues (see below).

The effects of direct current application to the body

The following explains why specific treatments are effective. Therapists who do not require such details should proceed to the sections on specific treatments where the appropriate effects are listed.

When a direct current is applied to the body certain effects are produced at the electrodes also known as 'poles'. These effects are known as 'polar effects'. Other effects are produced in the tissues between the electrodes or poles; these are known as 'interpolar effects'.

POLAR EFFECTS

These occur immediately beneath the electrodes.

ALKALINE REACTIONS

The production of the strong alkali, sodium hydroxide, at the cathode ($-$) is very irritating to the skin, and great care must be taken to avoid chemical burns to the skin (see page 124 regarding technique). The alkali saponifies the sebum and has a drying effect on the skin. It breaks down the keratin in keratinised cells, thus softening the skin and scar tissue. It neutralises the acidity of the skin, destroying the acid mantle and, therefore, reducing its germicidal properties.

ACID REACTIONS

The production of hydrochloric acid at the anode ($+$) also has an irritating effect, but is less marked than at the cathode. It can, however, cause burns to the skin, but these will differ in appearance from burns produced under the cathode.

The tissues under the anode tend to tighten, harden and improve in condition – this is due to the hardening effect of the acid and also to the release of oxygen which will nourish and improve the vitality of the cells. The production of acid increases the acidic protection of the skin and increases its germicidal properties.

VASODILATION

The irritating nature of the alkali and acid at the poles produces vasodilation under both electrodes. It is more marked and lasts longer under the cathode due to greater irritation. Vasodilation occurs because skin reacts to irritation by a process known as the 'triple response'.

Firstly, irritation of the cells causes release of histamine – this results in dilation of the capillaries, producing erythema or reddening of the skin.

Secondly, further reddening is produced by 'axon reflex', which produces dilation of arterioles in the area. Nerve impulses travelling from pain receptors through the axon can travel directly through another axon branch to the arterial wall without proceeding to the central nervous system. These impulses stimulate the muscle wall of the artery to relax and the vessel to dilate.

Thirdly, more severe irritation will result in increased permeability of capillary walls and plasma will pass out into the tissues. This will increase the amount of tissue fluid in the area. It can be seen that the irritation under the electrodes will produce vasodilation giving hyperaemia, erythema and heat.

Figure 6.3 *Impulses transmitted from sensory receptor directly to the arteriol wall resulting in dilation*

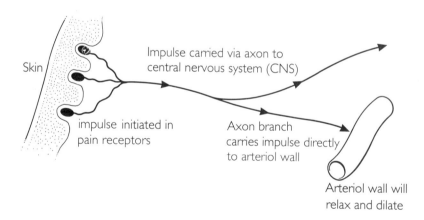

These effects are far greater under the cathode (−) due to the intense irritating quality of sodium hydroxide and the release of active hydrogen.

PRODUCTION OF HEAT

An increase in blood flow to an area will raise the temperature of the area. During galvanic treatments, the degree of heat produced will be directly proportional to the intensity of the current, the time for which it flows and the resistance offered to the current.

Again the heating under the cathode (−) is greater than under the anode (+) due to greater vasodilation.

Particular attention must be paid to technique when applying galvanic treatments in order to minimise any risk of causing thermal burns, (see page 121).

EXCITABILITY OF NERVES

The cathode (−) reduces the resting potential difference (PD) of a nerve, thus increasing conductivity and excitability. The anode (+) increases the resting PD of the nerve thus reducing conductivity and excitability. Prolonged treatment may result in numbing of the area – an analgesic effect at the anode.

FLUID CONTENT

There is an increase in tissue fluid under the cathode (−) – this is partly due to the increased permeability of vessel walls and also because water molecules move away from the anode (+) towards the cathode (−). This effect can be used to soften scars.

THE EFFECTS OF REPELLING IONS INTO THE SKIN (IONTOPHORESIS) WILL BE SPECIFIC TO THE TYPE OF MANUFACTURED PRODUCT SELECTED

Many products are produced in different forms, eg gels, ampules and serums, for the treatment of various conditions. The manufacturer's instructions must be carefully read and adhered to and the correct electrode must be selected to repel the ions in the gel. Like charges repel, therefore, if the gel contains negatively charged beneficial ions, the cathode (−) must be used as the active electrode.

If the gel contains positively charged beneficial ions, then the anode (+) is used as the active electrode.

The inactive electrode is placed elsewhere on the body to complete the circuit.

INTERPOLAR EFFECTS

In addition to the effects immediately under the poles, there are effects in the tissues between the electrodes.

BLOOD CIRCULATION

There is an increase in blood circulating through the tissues. Therefore, nutrients and oxygen are brought to the area and metabolites are removed more quickly.

LYMPHATIC CIRCULATION

There is an increase in lymphatic circulation, thus removing waste products more quickly.

INCREASED CELL METABOLISM

There is an increase in the permeability of cell walls resulting in increased cell metabolism. Chemical compounds within the cells are split into ions making them easier to remove.

REDUCTION IN BLOOD PRESSURE

Body galvanic treatments reduce both diastolic and systolic pressure. This should be borne in mind if clients suffer from low blood pressure.

Machines, galvanic units and systems

There is a wide variety of machines on the market for use as facial units, body units and combined facial and body units. Low voltage direct current is produced by a battery or modified AC mains. This current is applied to the body using electrodes connected to the machine by leads. One electrode will be negative called the cathode. The other will be positive called the anode. All machines have intensity controls and a milliammeter to indicate current flow. Machines may have single sockets for each pair of leads (ie each connecting jack will divide into two leads) *or* the machine may have independent sockets for each lead. In this instance, the connectors on the machine are usually coloured red or black.

If the unit has independent colour sockets for each lead (often used in facial systems), the red and black connecting leads must be plugged into matching coloured sockets. Units with single sockets have a red or black pin to identify polarity.

Both facial and body systems usually include a polarity reversal switch. This is intended to reverse the polarity should the therapist require to do so during the treatment. Because machines are not standardised, the polarity switch may be misinterpreted by the therapist and this can lead to incorrect treatment. It is vital to refer to each individual manufacturer's instruction manual to ensure understanding and correct use of machine.

EXAMPLES OF WORDING AND SWITCHING FOUND ON DIFFERENT UNITS

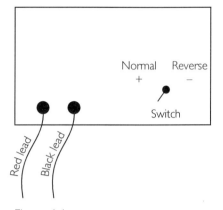

Figure 6.4

On this unit, the polarity indicator uses two types of instructions; symbols ('+' and '−') and wording ('normal' and 'reverse'). Manufacturers will consider the wording 'normal' and 'reverse' to automatically indicate the *normal* law of colour coding (ie red = positive and black = negative).

When the switch is moved to positive, the red lead is positive (+). When switched to negative the red lead is negative (−).

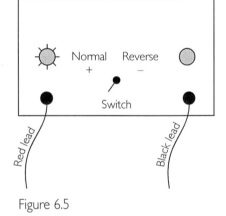

Figure 6.5

Some manufacturers help to make the polarity switch more visually obvious. The ISIS module galvanic has independent connecting plugs as above and the red and black leads plug in as normal.

When the switch is moved to the left, the normal position, a red light illuminates the red connector indicating that this connector is positive. When the switch is moved to the right (ie reverse), a red light illuminates the black connector indicating that this has now become the positive connector.

The greatest confusion arises when using a single socket outlet. The two leads may be coloured (one red and one black) or may be buff coloured with the terminal ends coloured (one red, one black).

If the polarity switch uses only symbols as above, it is essential to read the manufacturer's instructions to establish how the system has been designed as the switch could be wired in two different ways.

I On some machines, the design may be such that when the switch is set to the '+' symbol, the red terminal is the positive (+) and the black terminal is the negative (−). When the switch is set to the '−' symbol, the red becomes negative (−) and the black becomes positive (+). This is fairly straightforward as the red lead is thought of as the master lead.
But:

Figure 6.6

Figure 6.7

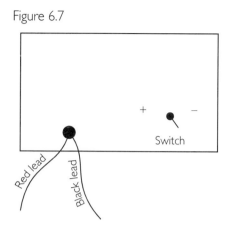

2 On other machines, when the switch is flicked towards the '−', then the black lead is negative (−) and the red lead is positive (+). By reversing the switch the black lead has become positive (+) and the red lead negative (−).

This can lead to a great deal of confusion; therefore, always check with the manufacturer's instructions.

It is always vital to check the polarity output of each machine oneself. To check the polarity, hold both electrodes in your hand and increase the intensity; the negative electrode/pole will always be the more irritating. This test is the easiest to perform, but is not as definite as the water test. Hold the leads in a beaker of water and increase the intensity; bubbles of hydrogen will be seen at the cathode (−). Red litmus paper could also be used – this will turn blue under the cathode.

Figure 6.8   *If electrodes are immersed in saline solution or water, bubbles of hydrogen gas will show at the cathode when the current is switched on*

Students must always ensure that they understand all the components on the machines in order to give effective treatments. Older machines are still found in some departments and salons. These will differ in design and may have a 'shunt' switch. This switch, when moved from 0 to 10, will multiply the current by 10. Therefore, on the meter:

- A reading of 1 mA indicates an output of 10 mA
- A reading of 2 mA indicates an output of 20 mA

These current intensities are far too high and great care must be taken if using these machines.

The terminology applied to the electrodes is also confusing. One electrode will always be negatively charged, called the cathode. The other will be positively charged, called the anode. Normal colour coding indicates that the cathode is black and the anode is red, but as previously explained, this may not always apply.

Various names are also used when describing the electrode which is producing the required effect and the one merely completing the circuit:

| Active | – Passive | Active | – Indifferent |
| Active | – Inactive | Differential | – Passive |

Facial disincrustation treatment

The direct or galvanic current is used in two ways on the face to improve cleanliness, tone texture and condition of the skin. The methods are known as disincrustation and iontophoresis.

Disincrustation treatment is based on *the chemistry of electrolysis* and uses the chemical reaction produced when a direct current is passed through saline solution (see page 100).

The alkali, sodium hydroxide, formed under the cathode (−) will soften the build up of sebum, breakdown keratinised cells of the superficial layer of the skin, open pores and release blockages. It is, therefore, used as a general and deep cleansing treatment.

The treatment requires a source of direct current applied to the body via two electrodes, a cathode (−) which must be the active electrode and an anode (+) which is the inactive electrode. It also requires a salt solution as an electrolyte (made by mixing 2 teaspoonfuls of salt to 1 litre of water). There are manufactured products available which produce the same effect but will be more costly.

Figure 6.9   *A facial galvanic unit with electrodes*

ELECTRODES

The anode (+) is the inactive electrode and must be placed in a comfortable position on the client to complete the circuit. It may be a metal rod, which is held in the client's hand, or a metal plate, which is placed on the upper arm. In both cases, it must be covered with moist lint or dense foam which must be of even texture 1 cm or $\frac{1}{2}$ inch thick and larger by 1 cm or $\frac{1}{2}$ inch than the electrode.

The cathode (−) is the active electrode and is the one used on the face for disincrustation treatments. There are several varieties:

1 disc electrode;
2 tweezer electrode;
3 mask electrode.

USES AT THE CATHODE (−)

1 General cleansing of a combination and greasy skin.
2 Deep cleansing of a seborrhoeic skin.
3 Stimulation of a sluggish skin with build up of keratinised cells and comedomes.

A careful skin analysis must be carried out before treatment to ensure that the skin type is suitable for disincrustation. Although fluid is temporarily drawn to the cathode (−), this treatment should not be used on a mature or dry/dehydrated skin as the caustic effect of the alkali, sodium hydroxide, would exacerbate the condition.

EFFECTS AT THE CATHODE (−)

1 The alkali, sodium hydroxide, formed will saponify sebum and soften the skin; the pores relax releasing the sebum. It will also break down the keratin in the superficial layers of the skin, thus softening and cleansing the area.
2 Fluid drawn towards the cathode (−) will soften the skin. This hydrating effect is only temporary.
3 It causes vasodilation with hyperaemia and erythema; the increase in circulation brings nutrients and oxygen to nourish the skin and removes waste products. This will improve the condition of the skin and improve the colour of sallow sluggish skin.
4 It increases cell metabolism, which improves the condition of the skin.
5 The alkali, sodium hydroxide, alters the pH of the skin, destroying the acid mantle. This is an undesirable effect and is

corrected by reversing the polarity at the end of the treatment
for 2–4 minutes.

EFFECTS AT THE ANODE (+) (WHEN THE POLARITY IS REVERSED)

1 The formation of hydrochloric acid restores the acid mantle.
2 The acid tightens and firms the skin.
3 Tissue fluid moves away from the anode.
4 There is little vasodilation with erythema.
5 The release of oxygen revitalises the tissues.

USES AT THE ANODE (+)

The effects at the anode (+) can be used to improve the tone and
texture of the skin and refine a skin with large, open pores. The
hydrochloric acid formed will tighten the tissue and help to close
the pores. It will restore the acid mantle and improve the skin's
resistance to infection. The oxygen will help to nourish and
revitalise the tissues.

CONTRA-INDICATIONS

1 Lack of skin sensitivity, which may be caused by damage to or
  pressure on nerves, neurological disorders, scarring. Bell's palsy
  or dental treatments, etc. (Always check with hot and cold and
  with blunt and sharp tests (see page 111).
2 Cuts and abrasions (cover small cuts with petroleum jelly and
  plaster).
3 Metal pins or plates around the head or excessive fillings.
4 Hypersensitive skins, eg rosacea, dermatitis and telangiectasis.
5 Pustular acne with inflamed areas.
6 Highly nervous clients.

DANGERS

1 *Burns.* The danger of burns with facial galvanic correctly applied
  is minimal as the time of application is short, current intensity
  low and the electrode is moving continually.
2 *Shock.* There is danger of shock if the current is turned up or
  down suddenly, if the electrodes are lifted off the skin during
  treatment or if the resistance of the skin drops suddenly.

PRECAUTIONS

1 Check for contra-indications.
2 Test for skin sensitivity.
3 Check that all jewellery has been removed.

4 Check the machine and test it on yourself.

5 Ensure that salt crystals have dissolved.

6 Saturate the gauze or pad evenly.

7 Place the active electrode on a sensitive area, such as the forehead, and turn the current up very slowly.

8 Keep the pad moist during treatment (use a dropper if necessary).

9 Turn the current down slowly before lifting the electrode.

10 Speak to the client throughout the treatment.

Figure 6.10   *Disincrustation treatment*

TREATMENT TECHNIQUE

PREPARATION OF THE CLIENT

1 Place the client in a well-supported and comfortable position.

2 Check that all jewellery has been removed.

3 Check for contra-indications.

4 Explain the treatment to the client.

5 Cleanse and tone the skin.

6 Check for sensitivity to hot and cold. Use two test tubes, one containing hot water and one containing cold water. Tell the client to close her eyes. Touch randomly over the face with the hot and cold test tubes asking the client to identify which one is touching her. Also test her sensitivity to blunt and sharp using an orange stick/blunt needle and cotton wool (proceed as for hot and cold). If the client is able to identify both hot/cold and blunt/sharp, her sensation is intact and the treatment may proceed. If she is unable to repeatedly identify either, her sensation is defective and treatment should not be carried out.

7 Apply a little petroleum jelly around the eye to prevent 'flash'. (This is an uncomfortable feeling which may happen if the electrode moves too near the eye.)

PROCEDURE

1 Position the machine on a stable base and check that the plugs, leads and terminals are secure and away from water.
2 Check that the intensity control is at zero.
3 Collect all commodities.
4 Test the machine: hold both electrodes in one hand and increase the intensity of the current.
5 Prepare a saline solution – stir 2 teaspoonfuls of salt into 1 litre of water; make sure that all the crystals have dissolved. (Or select disincrustation gel if this is to be used.)
6 Select the appropriate electrodes and plug them into the machine.
7 Saturate all lint or sponges in saline solution: if you are using a gauze mask, saturate this; if you are using a manufacturer's gel, apply this thinly and evenly over greasy areas of the face, or use it to saturate the gauze.
8 Place a dampened cover around the inactive electrode (anode) and give it to the client to hold if it is a rod elecrrode, or strap it on to the upper arm if it is a plate electrode.
9 Secure the saturated gauze/lint to the active electrode (the cathode (−)).
10 Explain the sensation to the client and ask her to report any discomfort.
11 Place the cathode on the client's skin. Choose an area of high sensitivity, eg the forehead, and switch on.
12 Turn the current up slowly moving the electrode on the face. Very low current is needed, up to a maximum of 2 mA. This must be within the client's tolerance.
13 As soon as the client feels a prickling sensation, turn the current down slightly.
14 Move the electrode slowly over face and neck using a circular movement. Cover the face or greasy areas evenly for up to 10 minutes or according to manufacturer's instructions.
15 At the end of the treatment turn the intensity down very slowly and switch off with electrode still in contact with the face.
16 Replace the lint or gauze and reverse the polarity of the machine.
17 Place the electrode on the face again and repeat the procedure for 2–5 minutes. (This will restore the pH of the skin.)
18 Turn the intensity down slowly as before and switch off.
19 The face must be thoroughly wiped over with damp cotton wool. Then apply toner and blot with tissue.
20 Clean the electrodes – wash them with hot water and detergent and wipe over with a disinfectant wipe.
   Make up should not be worn for 8 hours.

Facial iontophoresis

This uses a direct current to introduce beneficial products into the skin. The treatment is based on the principle that *like charges repel* and *opposite charges attract.*

A source of direct current is applied to the face or body and the electrodes are used to repel ions of beneficial substances into the skin.

Manufacturers produce a wide range of gels/serums, etc, suitable for various skin conditions. The products contain ions which carry either negative or positive charges. The success of this treatment is dependent upon:

1 Correct identification of the skin condition.
2 The selection of the appropriate product for the skin condition.
3 The selection of the appropriate electrode to repel the product. If the product is negatively charged, the cathode (−) will be the active electrode. The cathode (−) will repel the anions (−) in the product into the skin. If the product is positively charged, the anode (+) will be the active electrode. The anode (+) will repel the cations (+) in the product into the skin.

This movement of anions is called *anaphoresis* and the movement of cations is called *cataphoresis.*

Figure 6.11   *Galvanic unit with electrodes. The roller electrodes (1 and 2) are used as the active electrodes, 3 or 4 are used as the inactive.*

ELECTRODES

Types of electrode:

1 ball electrode;
2 roller electrode;
3 mask.

Gels and serums that are repelled under electrodes are thought to achieve deeper penetration than manual applications. Penetration is thought to be less than 1 mm, but deeper absorption may be achieved via the capillary circulation and transport through cell membranes.

Research has indicated that low level intensity currents and low ionic concentrations may well be as effective as high intensity currents and high ionic concentrations (on the basis that a few ions entering slowly will find it easier to enter the skin than a mass of ions all with the same charge repelling each other as they are forced through). However, some products may require certain intensities for their repulsion and manufacturers sometimes offer guidelines which should be carefully followed. When products without guidelines are used, it should be borne in mind that a low current is often effective.

USES

This form of treatment can be used for a wide variety of skin conditions. A careful skin analysis must be made to diagnose the problem areas. The appropriate product can then be selected to suit the needs of the client, eg:

1 *Hydration and moisturising*. Many products are manufactured for moisturising and hydrating a dry and mature skin; serums containing collagen, elastin and placental extracts are particularly beneficial.
2 *Regeneration*. Products are available for the repair and regeneration of mature skin and of damaged skin, particularly after exposure to the sun and wind.
3 *Stimulating*. Products for stimulating a sluggish, sallow complexion include extracts of seaweed and other marine products. Care must be taken not to over treat with these products.
4 *Improvement of sensitive skins*. Gels and serums are available for the treatment of the sensitive couperose skin. Care must be taken when treating these skin types as many conditions can be exacerbated by the direct current. Rosacea, dermatitis and highly vascular conditions would be contra-indicated and should not be treated with galvanic current.

EFFECTS

1 When using iontophoresis the main effect will depend on, and be specific to, the product used. Manufacturers recommend their products for specific skin types and also indicate which electrode should be used for repelling the ions into the skin.

The products come in many forms (eg gels, ampules, serums, impregnated gauze etc.) and contain extracts of beneficial substance such as collagen, elastin, placental or herbal extracts of ivy, seaweed etc. Therefore careful skin analysis must be carried out and the appropriate product selected to achieve the most effective beneficial outcome for the client. Other effects will be due to stimulation by the direct current.

2 Vasodilation, with hyperaemia and erythema, will increase the circulation to the face bringing oxygen and nutrients to improve the condition of the skin.

3 The increase in cell metabolism will improve the condition of the skin.

4 Desquamation is aided due to increase mitotic activity of the basal layer.

5 Improvement in the colour and texture of the skin due to an increase in blood flow and an increase in desquamation.

Contra-indications

1 Lack of skin sensitivity.
2 Cuts and abrasions.
3 Metal pins or plates.
4 Hypersensitive skins, eg rosacea, dermatitis and telangiectasis.
5 Pustular acne with inflamed areas.
6 Highly nervous clients.

Dangers

1 *Burns.* The danger of burns is minimal as the rollers are continually moving and the current intensity is low.
2 *Shock.* There is a danger of shock if the current is turned up or down suddenly, or if the intensity is turned up before the electrode is in contact with the face, or if the rollers knock together during treatment.

Precautions

1 Test the client's skin sensitivity with hot/cold, blunt/sharp.
2 Check that the controls are at zero.
3 Test the current on yourself.
4 Apply the gel or ampule content evenly and thinly over the face. If using a gauze mask, saturate it evenly and make sure that it is applied smoothly to the face with no wrinkling or puckering.
5 Place the rollers on a sensitive area of skin, eg the forehead or jaw line, and keep them moving while turning the current up slowly and steadily.

6 Turn the intensity down slightly when the client feels a tingling sensation. (Remember this treatment is more effective with a low intensity current and low ionic concentrations. Turn the current up only within the tolerance of the client.)

7 Move the rollers slowly over the face without breaking contact with the skin.

8 Do not knock the rollers together during treatment.

9 Turn the current down slowly before removing the electrodes.

10 Do not allow the skin to become dry during treatment as the treatment would become ineffective.

11 Use petroleum jelly around the eyes. This acts as insulation to prevent 'flash'.

12 Always follow manufacturers' instructions for the timing of the treatment.

13 Speak to the client throughout the treatment.

TREATMENT TECHNIQUE

Figure 6.12   *Iontophoresis treatment*

PREPARATION OF THE CLIENT

1 Place the client in a well-supported and comfortable position.

2 Check that all jewellery has been removed.

3 Check for contra-indications.

4 Explain the treatment to the client.

5 Cleanse and tone the skin.

6 Check for skin sensitivity with hot and cold test tubes and an orange stick and cotton wool (see page 111).

7 Apply petroleum jelly around the eye to prevent flash (see page 111).

8 Select the appropriate gel, serum, etc, to suit the skin type and check its charge, ie negative or positive.

PROCEDURE

1 Position the machine on a stable base and check that the plugs leads and terminals are secure.

2 Check that the intensity control is at zero.

3 Select the active roller electrodes and plug them into the machine: negative if the gel is negatively charged; positive if the gel is positively charged.

4 Plug in the inactive electrode into the other socket.

5 Test the machine, hold the active and inactive electrodes in one hand and increase the intensity of the current.

6 Cover the inactive electrode with moistened foam or lint $\frac{1}{2}$ inch thick and give it to the client to hold, or strap it on to upper arm if it is a plate electrode.

7 Apply gel or the contents of the ampule thinly and evenly over the face and neck, or place saturated gauze over the face and neck.

8 Check that the controls are at zero.

9 Place one roller on to the client's skin, switch on the machine and turn up the current slowly until a tingling sensation is felt, then place the other roller on the other side.

10 Move the rollers over the face without breaking contact with the skin and making sure the rollers do not touch each other. Maintain an even pressure and a slow, rhythmical movement.

11 Ask the client to report any discomfort.

12 Remove one roller and turn the current down slowly and switch off the current before removing the other roller.

13 If necessary, apply a little more gel on the chin and nose and use single ball or fork electrode for concentrated work.

14 Remove excess gel, tone and moisturiser. Do not apply make up for 8 hours.

15 Clean the electrodes – wash them with hot water and detergent, dry and wipe them with a disinfectant wipe.

Note: It is the tolerance of the client which dictates the maximum current from 0.05 mA–2 mA.

High frequency and facial galvanic treatments may be combined to offer effective facial routines.

Figure 6.13 (a, b, c)   *High frequency and facial galvanic treatment*

Body galvanism

The application of a direct current to the tissues of the body will produce certain physiological effects (see page 102). These effects are thought to soften areas of fat or cellulite and aid its dispersal. There are various ways in which the galvanic current is used to produce these effects.

1 The traditional method of applying the direct current uses electrodes covered with pads soaked in saline solution. This method uses the polar and interpolar effect and is generally called body galvanism.

   The most irritating and stimulating effects produced at the cathode (−) are used in this method. Therefore the cathode (−) is always the active electrode and is placed over the areas of cellulite while the anode (+) is always placed opposite it or in parallel with it as the inactive electrode.

2 The more modern method uses anti-cellulite gels and ampules containing liquid serum preparations specially manufactured to treat cellulite. These preparations contain charged ions of beneficial substances which are repelled into the skin by use of the appropriate electrode. The gel usually carries negatively charged beneficial ions; therefore, the cathode (−) is used to repel them into the tissues. However, if it carries a positive charge, the anode (+) must be used; always check with the manufacturer's instructions. This method uses the effects of the gel as well as some of the polar and the interpolar effects of the current. This form of treatment is known as body iontophoresis.

3 Certain modern systems utilise the galvanic current in the

Figure 6.14 *A galvanic unit showing body electrodes, pads and strapping*

treatment of the whole body, via body wraps, clay etc. These treatments use specially formulated products to achieve the desired results. The current is used for its effect in stimulating the circulation, increasing lymphatic drainage and for stimulating metabolic rate, thus enhancing the effect of the products. These treatments use far lower current intensities than the previous methods, and manufacturer's instructions must be strictly adhered to.

USES

1 To soften areas of fat/cellulite and aid its absorption.
2 To stimulate the circulation of blood and lymph, thus improving the condition of the skin and tissues.
3 To improve areas of stasis.
4 Body galvanism can be used to soften areas of old, hard scar tissue. The cathode must be used for this as fluid is attracted to the cathode.

SUMMARY OF EFFECTS

(For a full explanation, see p 102.)

POLAR EFFECTS UNDER THE CATHODE (−) (ACTIVE ELECTRODE):

1 The alkali, sodium hydroxide, is formed. This softens the skin and tissues.
2 Hydrogen is released which is stimulating to the tissues.
3 Vasodilation with hyperaemia and erythema; more blood will flow to the area bringing nutrients and oxygen and removing metabolites.
4 Irritation of sensory nerve endings; it increases the conductivity of nerves.
5 An increase in the water and tissue fluid in the area of the electrode due to increased permeability of vessel walls and to the movement of water molecules away from the anode (+) towards the cathode (−). This will soften the area.
6 Heat is produced under the electrode; the client should feel an even, comfortable warmth.
7 Products, such as gels and ampules, containing negatively charged ions will be repelled into the skin by the cathode (−). The effect produced will be specific to that product, eg anti-cellulite products will aid breakdown and dispersal of cellulite.

POLAR EFFECTS UNDER THE ANODE (+)

The anode is usually the inactive electrode in body galvanism. Its effects are not utilised in the treatment:

1 Hydrochloric acid is formed, which tightens and hardens the skin and tissues.
2 Oxygen is released which increases the vitality of the tissues.
3 Vasodilation with hyperaemia and erythema result, but this is not as great as under the cathode (−).
4 It decreases the conductivity of nerves and may have an analgesic effect under the pad.
5 A decrease in water content as water molecules move away from the anode (+) towards the cathode (−).
6 Heat is produced under the electrode.
7 Products containing positively charged ions will be repelled into the skin by the anode (+).

INTERPOLAR EFFECTS

1 An increase in circulation.
2 An increase in metabolic rate.
3 An increase in lymphatic drainage.
4 The lowering of blood pressure.

CONTRA-INDICATIONS

1 Lack of skin sensitivity may be due to neurological disorders, injury, scar tissue, etc.
2 Cuts or abrasions; small cuts can be covered with petroleum jelly and waterproof plaster.
3 Extensive scar tissue.
4 Other skin conditions, such as eczema and psoriasis.
5 Metal pins or plates in the area to be treated.
6 Treatment around the abdomen must not be carried out on anyone with IUD coils.
7 Low blood pressure.
8 Pregnancy.
9 Any medication in the form of ointments that have been applied to the skin, such as Algipan, as these will sensitise the area. (Always wash skin thoroughly to avoid this possibility.)

DANGERS

The great danger with the application of direct current to the body is the production of burns, both chemical and, to a lesser extent, thermal. Burns are caused by poor technique of application and *must* be avoided (see page 124). An awareness of the nature and causes of galvanic burns will enable the therapist to develop good technique, thus ensuring that burns do not occur.

THERMAL BURNS

An increase in blood flow to an area will result in the production of heat to that area. The amount of heat produced will be directly proportional to the intensity, time and resistance. Because the processes of conduction, convection and radiation are restricted under the pads, there is a build up of heat.

Causes of thermal burns
If the intensity of the current is high, the time during which it flows is too long or if the resistance to the current is high, there is a danger of producing a thermal burn. The intensity and time of current flow must be carefully controlled and careful consideration must be given to avoid areas of high resistance. Care must be taken to avoid large freckles and areas of hard tissue, such as scars. If scars are being treated, the current intensity must be kept very low below 2 mA.

The most common causes of high resistance burns are: Pads being unevenly saturated, giving rise to dry/moist spots resulting in high areas of resistance (dry) and low areas of resistance (moist); unevenness within the pads preventing good even skin contact; gaps and air spaces allowed between the skin and the electrode. This happens if a stiff electrode does not adapt to the rounded contour of the body.

Burns may also occur if the client is lying with full body weight on the electrode. This pressure limits the circulating blood and its action of conducting heat away from the area. Therefore, if the posterior aspect of the body is being treated, clients should lie in the prone position (face down) and vice versa.

Tight rubber bandages also produce ischaemic conditions; they should apply even firm pressure over the electrode but not be so tight as to occlude the circulation.

CHEMICAL BURNS

There is a greater risk of chemical burns than heat burns, and the risk is greater under the cathode ($-$) than under the anode ($+$) because the strong alkali, sodium hydroxide, causes destruction and softening of the tissues. A red sore mark appears immediately, and this later changes to a grey oozing wound. These wounds take a long time to heal and should be treated with care. Cover with a dry, sterile dressing taking care that it does not become infected.

Burns under the anode (+) are more rare due to the low concentration of hydrochloric acid. The skin under the anode (+) will be dryer and tougher and the burn appears as a hardened lump or scab. It should be treated with care in the same way as above. There are many causes of chemical burns; they are all the result of undue care and lack of attention to detail. Therapists must develop a good technique to avoid these complications.

Causes of chemical burns

Chemical burns may occur for the following reasons:

1 If the intensity of the current is too high and if the treatment time is too long – these will cause greater concentrations of both sodium hydroxide at the cathode (−) and hydrochloric acid at the anode (+).
2 If the current concentrates on one area. This may be due to:
   (a) a break in the skin;
   (b) the pads being unevenly folded and of uneven thickness;
   (c) the pads being unevenly moistened or containing undissolved salt;
   (d) the electrode or its connections coming into direct contact with the skin.
3 If the current is applied with metal touching the tissues, either in the form of jewellery, or metal plates and pins in tissues, or IUD coils. Always remove jewellery and avoid giving treatment to areas around metal plates and IUD coils.
4 If the pads are too close so that current concentrates between them.
5 If the pads are too thin, the acid and alkali will not be absorbed and dissipated.
6 If the chemicals have not been washed out of the pads after a previous treatment.
7 If the client has defective skin sensation and is unable to feel that the intensity is too high or that the current is concentrating in one spot.
8 If the treatment has not been explained carefully to the client. (The importance of reporting discomfort and hot spots and the consequences of not doing so must be explained clearly to the client.)

SHOCK

There is a danger of shock to the client:

1 If the apparatus is faulty and monitoring controls are not functioning and operating correctly.

2 If the current intensity is increased too quickly or reduced suddenly.

3 If skin resistance drops suddenly. As the skin becomes moist, the resistance to the current is lowered. Modern equipment will adjust automatically to a fall in skin resistance and the current intensity will reduce accordingly. However, when using the older constant voltage machines, the current intensity must be reduced manually as the skin resistance falls. Therefore, the apparatus must be checked before treatment.

PRECAUTIONS

1 Check for contra-indications.
2 Test for skin sensitivity.
3 Check that all jewellery has been removed.
4 Wash the area thoroughly.
5 Check the machine and test it on yourself; ensure the intensity controls are at zero.
6 If using a saline solution, mix 2 teaspoonfuls of salt per litre of warm water; make sure that all the crystals have dissolved.
7 Prepare the pads. They must be of even thickness and not worn or cracked.
   (a) Measure the pads to calculate the current intensity, which should be 0.05 mA per square cm.
   (b) If using pre-made pads or sponge envelopes, ensure that they are of high density foam at least $\frac{1}{2}$ inch thick.
   (c) If using lint pads, carefully fold the sides to middle. Ensure that they are 16 layers and of even thickness, that they are smooth and contain no wrinkles or frayed edges.
   (d) Ensure that the pads are 1 cm/$\frac{1}{2}$ inch larger than the electrode all around.
   (e) Wash the pads in warm water to make absolutely sure that no chemicals remain in the pads from previous use.
8 Saturate the pads well and evenly. Wet and squeeze out any excess solution.
9 Mould the pad and electrode to the part, cover with insulating fabric and strap evenly and securely; ensure that there are no gaps between the skin and pad.
10 Turn the current up slowly; adjust if necessary.
11 At the end of the treatment, turn the current down slowly.
12 Speak to the client throughout the treatment.
13 Wash the area thoroughly with warm soapy water after treatment to remove chemical build up on the skin.
14 Wash the pads in warm soapy water, rinse and hang to dry.

Figure 6.15   *Method of applying lint pad* →

Figure 6.16   *Method of applying sponge envelopes* →

Figure 6.17   *To calculate the intensity of the current required for body treatment measure two sides of the pad (one long and one short) multiply these, to obtain the number of square centimetres. Each square centimetre of pad should receive 0·05 milliamps of current, therefore multiply the number of square centimetres by 0·05 milliamps. Therefore for this size of pad the maximum anchorage would be eight milliamps.* →

TREATMENT TECHNIQUE

PREPARATION OF THE CLIENT

1 Consider the areas to be treated and position the client accordingly. If the thighs and hips are to be treated, place the client in the supine position (face up). If the buttocks or back are to be treated, place the client in the prone position (face down).

2 Check that all jewellery has been removed.

3 Check for contra-indications.

4 Check particularly for broken skin, eg cuts and abrasions, as they offer low resistance to current; therefore, the current would concentrate here and cause a burn. Small cuts can be insulated with petroleum jelly and covered with waterproof plasters.

5 Test skin sensitivity with hot and cold test tubes and a blunt needle and cotton wool (see page 111).

6 Wash the area thoroughly to remove sweat, moisturisers, lotions, perfumes, etc.

7 Explain the treatment to the client.

PROCEDURE

1 Place the machine on a stable base and check that the plugs, electrodes, leads and terminals are sound and secure.

2 Check that the intensity controls are at zero, and if there is a shunt (which multiplies the intensity by ten) move this to the low point.

3 Test the machine.

4 Collect all the prepared items mentioned previously and have them to hand.

5 Wash the pads in warm water and then either wet them in saline solution and squeeze out the excess or, if using gels, etc, soak them with water and squeeze out the excess.

6 If a gel or ampule is used, either apply this directly to the area ensuring an even application, or soak into a piece of gauze and apply this to the skin ensuring a smooth, even contact.

7 Place the electrode over the pad (or in a pouch) making sure than the pad is $\frac{1}{2}$ inch bigger all around, and is $\frac{1}{2}$ inch deep. (The pad must lie between the skin and the electrode.)

8 Place the active electrode over the treatment area and the inactive electrode opposite or parallel to it. Mould them to the body. If using a saline solution the cathode ($-$) will be the active electrode. If using products, follow the manufacturer's instructions. If the product contains negative anions, the cathode ($-$) will be the active electrode, but if the product contains positive cations, the anode ($+$) will be the active electrode.

9 Cover both electrodes with insulating fabric (rubber, plastic or polythene). There must be no holes in this. This is so that the connective straps do not become conductive.

10 Secure the pad and insulating fabric evenly in position with straps (make sure the electrodes mould to the body and contain no air spaces and that strapping applies even pressure all over).

11 Explain the sensation to the client and stress the importance of reporting any discomfort, any concentration of current in one area or any hot spots. The client should feel a slight tingling sensation which will give way to *mild* warmth.

12 Check that the electrodes have not moved.

13 Turn up the intensity control very slowly until a sensation of warmth is felt. The desired intensity will depend on the clients' tolerance, product usage and size of the pad. Most products and client comfort indicate 0.05 mA per sq cm.

14 Stay with the client; as the treatment progresses, the skin resistance will fall. Some machines that are designed as constant voltage will register an increase in intensity as the skin resistance falls. With this type of machine, the intensity will

need to be turned down accordingly. Most modern systems are designed as constant current, and will automatically adjust to changes in body resistance.

15 The treatment should last for 20 minutes; at the end of treatment, turn the intensity control down very slowly. (A sudden increase or decrease in current intensity gives the client a shock, as the muscles may contract.)

16 The skin should be evenly pink under each pad, and there should be a more marked reaction under the cathode ($-$).

17 If using saline, wash the skin thoroughly with warm, soapy water and dry gently. This will remove any acid or alkali. Apply a soothing lotion or talc.

18 Wash the pads thoroughly in soapy water, rinse and leave them to dry.

Note: Do not carry out any other treatment over the area of the skin under the pads, as it is very sensitive.

SUGGESTION FOR BODY PADDING

Figure 6.18 (a, b, c, d)   *Body galvanic – suggested methods for padding. N = negative electrode and P = positive electrode.*

(a) Full body padding – anterior

(b) Full body padding – posterior

(c) Leg padding – parallel padding

(d) Leg padding – opposite padding

COMBINED SYSTEMS

Body wraps, clays, combined EMS and galvanic treatments. These treatments require specialised tuition from the manufacturers as each system differs in terms of application. Therapists must ensure that they attend courses and read the manufacturer's instructions carefully before embarking on these treatments.

Figure 6.19   *Client receiving body wrap treatment*

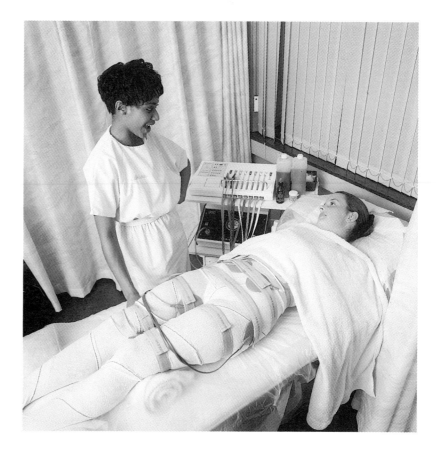

SUMMARY

- Galvanic treatments use a low voltage direct (or constant) current, sometimes called a galvanic current. This current flows in one direction only and has polarity.
- One electrode is negatively charged, called the *cathode*, the other electrode is positively charged, called the *anode*.
- Treatments which use the direct current are:

  Disincrustation – facial treatment – cleansing.

  Iontophoresis – facial treatment – beneficial ions for various skin types.

Body galvanism – body cellulite using sodium chloride solution.

Body iontophoresis – body cellulite using products.

- There is a variety of other body systems utilizing, clays, wraps, etc (epilation is not covered in this book).

- The effects produced depend on two scientific principles: the chemistry of electrolysis, and the law of physics which states that like charges repel (ie positive repels positive and negative repels negative) and opposite charges attract (ie positive attracts negative).

- Electrolyte is a solution which transmits a current. The compounds making up the solution dissociate (split) into cations (+) and anions (−). These move towards opposite poles because of the attraction of opposite charges. Therefore: *cations* (+) move towards the *cathode* (−), and *anions* (−) move towards the *anode* (+). Certain chemical reactions take place at the electrodes.

- When using sodium chloride solution (salt and water), the reactions at the electrodes will produce: sodium hydroxide (alkali) and hydrogen gas at the cathode and hydrochloric acid and oxygen gas at the anode.

DISINCRUSTATION TREATMENT TO THE FACE

- This uses lint soaked in sodium chloride or other products over the active electrode. When the current is flowing, the alkali, sodium hydroxide, is produced at the cathode. This alkali will saponify sebum, break down keratin, relax pores, releasing blockages and sebum which will soften and cleanse the skin.

- Its disadvantages are that it has a very drying effect and that it destroys the acid mantle. If the polarity is reversed at the end of the treatment, the hydrochloric acid produced restores the acid mantle.

IONTOPHORESIS

- This is the repulsion of ions of beneficial substances into the skin. These substances must be placed under the correct electrode for repulsion to take place. If the product contains negative *anions*, the negative *cathode* must be used for repulsion (anion active). If the product contains positive *cations*, the positive *anode* must be used for repulsion (cation active). Remember, like charges repel.

- This is a very effective and useful treatment as a wide variety of products are available to treat most skin types.

- There is very little danger with facial work, as the current intensities are low and the electrodes are moving. However, the client will receive a shock if the intensity is turned up or down too quickly, or if the electrode is lifted off the skin with the intensity turned up. This is because the sudden surge of current will stimulate the muscles to contract. This will also happen if the electrodes touch each other during iontophoresis treatment.

- The intensity of the current used for facial work will depend on the tolerance of the client and the erythema reaction produced. From 0.05–2 mA maximum is recommended by most manufacturers.

- It is essential to establish that the client is able to feel heat or sharp touch so that she can report any feeling of discomfort (for both facial and body work). Failure to report these sensations may result in burns. Test over the area receiving treatment with a hot and a cold test tube and with sharp and blunt instruments (an orange stick and some cotton wool are suitable). The client must close her eyes and identify which item is in contact with her skin.

BODY GALVANISM

- This uses pads soaked in saline solution. The active electrode is the *cathode* (−). The inactive electrode is placed opposite it or parallel with it.

- The effects are produced by the formation of irritating sodium hydroxide and hydrogen at the *cathode* and by changes in circulation, metabolic rate and water content of the tissue through which the current passes. It is used to reduce and soften areas of cellulite.

BODY IONTOPHORESIS

- This uses a gel or liquid anti-cellulite preparation placed under the appropriate electrode: negative under the *cathode* and positive under the *anode.* This substance will be repelled into the skin to produce the desired effect. There will also be changes in the circulation and metabolic rate of the tissue through which the current passes.

BODY SYSTEMS WHICH APPLY SPECIALLY MANUFACTURED SERUMS, ETC, VIA WRAPS AND CLAYS TO THE WHOLE OR LARGE PARTS OF THE BODY

- These use very low intensity current to stimulate the circulation.

DANGERS

Chemical burns, thermal burns and electric shock.

CHECK LIST

All students should ensure that they have checked and carried out all the following points of technique.

1 Make the client comfortable in a suitable position.
2 Remove all jewellery, any metal or water from the area.
3 Test for skin sensitivity – hot/cold; blunt/sharp.
4 Check for contra-indications.
5 Wash the area thoroughly.
6 Check that the machine and all plugs, leads, electrodes and terminals are sound and secure.
7 Ensure that the intensity controls are at zero.
8 Prepare the pads – ensuring that they are;
   (a) of even texture and density
   (b) folded evenly – no wrinkles or frayed edges
   (c) 1 cm or $\frac{1}{2}$ inch thick, $\frac{1}{2}$ inch larger than the electrode all around.
9 Mix a saline solution; 2 teaspoons of salt to 1 litre of warm water. Make sure all the salt has dissolved.
10 Wet pads and squeeze out the excess. If using a gel or lotion, soak a piece of gauze or apply thinly and evenly over the skin under active electrode.
11 Select the *cathode* (−) as the active electrode and the *anode* (+) as the inactive electrode (unless the product carries a positive charge).
12 Position the pad, electrode and waterproof insulating fabric.
13 Secure evenly and firmly with strapping; mould to the part leaving no air gaps.
14 Explain the sensation to the client and impress upon her the importance of reporting any discomfort.
15 Turn the current intensity up *slowly*; watch the milliammeter and the client. (The intensity must be within the tolerance of the client – around 0.05 mA per sq cm of pad).
16 Stay with the client and turn down the intensity as the skin resistance falls if the machine does not automatically adjust.
17 At the end of the treatment time, approximately 20 minutes, turn the intensity down *slowly*.
18 Remove the pads.

19 Examine and wash the area thoroughly – apply talc or lotion.
20 Do not carry out further treatments over the area of skin under electrodes as it is very sensitive.
21 Wash the pads thoroughly, rinse and dry them.

QUESTIONS

1 Galvanic treatments use a direct current; explain briefly what is meant by direct current.

2 List the four treatments that use the direct current.

3 A direct current has polarity; give the name and charge of each pole.

4 When the compound sodium chloride dissolves in water it ionises into two ions; name the two ions and give their charge.

5 When a direct current is passed through saline (salt) solution, name:
(a) The alkali formed under the cathode.
(b) The acid formed under the anode.

6 Explain the terms 'active electrode' and 'inactive electrode'.

7 Which electrode would be selected as the active electrode for disincrustation treatments using a salt solution.

8 Give the skin type suitable for disincrustation treatments.

9 Explain briefly why the polarity of the electrodes may be changed for 2–5 minutes at the end of treatment.

10 Give the physical theories on which the treatment of iontophoresis depends.

11 Explain why the choice of products is very important when using iontophoresis treatments.

12 Give *four* contra-indications to facial galvanic treatments.

13 Give the function of the milliammeter.

14 How is the milliammeter calibrated?

15 On what factor does the selection of current intensity depend? Indicate the maximum current for facial work.

16 Body galvanism is given to improve areas of hard fat or cellulite. Give two reasons why it is effective.

17 Why do thin or uneven pads constitute a danger to the client?

18 Explain the importance of dissolving all the crystals of salt.

19 Why should one carry out a skin sensitivity test?

20 Explain the procedure for testing skin sensitivity.

21 Explain why the skin and the pads should be thoroughly washed after treatment.

22 Why might the current intensity increase slightly at the beginning of treatment although the control is not moved?

23 Explain the action to be taken if the current intensity increases (on older machines).

24 How would you instruct the client at commencement of treatment?

25 Briefly explain why the skin will be red at the end of a treatment.

CHAPTER 7

Radiation treatments

Figure 7.1   *A sunbed*

OBJECTIVES

After you have studied this chapter you will be able to:

1 Explain the terms wave length and frequency.
2 State the range wave lengths of ultraviolet and infrared rays.
3 Explain the principles of:
  (a) refraction;
  (b) reflection;
  (c) absorption.
4 Explain the following laws related to radiation:
  (a) law of Grotthus;
  (b) the cosine law;
  (c) the law of inverse squares.
5 Differentiate between the luminous and non-luminous lamps.
6 Explain the effects of infrared rays on body tissues.
7 List the contra-indications to infrared treatments.
8 Treat the client paying due consideration to maximum efficiency, comfort, safety and hygiene.
9 Differentiate between the three bands of ultraviolet light (UVL)
10 Explain the limit of penetration of each band.
11 Distinguish between the emission from high pressure mercury vapour lamps, overhead solariums and sunbeds.
12 Explain the effects of exposure to artificial sunlight.
13 List the contra-indications to use of sunbeds.
14 Explain the factors which determine the intensity of the reaction.
15 Treat the client, paying due consideration to maximum efficiency, comfort, safety and hygiene.
16 Explain the use and procedure for performing a patch test.
17 Explain the relationship between timing and distance when changing the distance of mercury vapour lamps.

Infrared irradiation for heating body tissues and ultraviolet irradiation for promoting tanning of the skin are the radiation treatments used in beauty therapy. Both infrared rays and ultraviolet rays are part of the electromagnetic spectrum.

The electromagnetic spectrum

The spectrum is made up of bands of radiation with differing wave lengths and frequencies, each of which will have different physiological effects on body tissues. It is thought that all electromagnetic rays are similar in form, being particles in motion. They are transverse waves which travel through space without the need of a conductor.

The speed, or velocity, at which they travel is the same for all the bands, being 300,000 km/sec (the speed of sound).

Wavelength

The bands of the electromagnetic spectrum have different wave lengths. The wave length is the distance between a point on one wave and the same point on the next wave.

Figure 7.2   *Wave length*

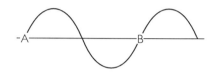

Wave length A to B

The distance from a to b is the wave length. This wave length varies from the very short wave length of cosmic rays, measured in nanometres, to the very long wave length of radio waves measured in metres or kilometres. (One nanometer is a very small measurement, being one millionth of a millimetre. It is written as nm.) The following table gives the wave lengths of each band emitted from the spectrum. There is overlap between some of the bands.

Table G *Wave lengths of each band emitted from the spectrum*

Short wave length					*Long wave length*	
			10 nm		400,000 nm	
Cosmic	Gamma	X-rays	Ultra-	Visible	Infra-	Radio
rays	rays		violet	light	red	
			Wave lengths utilised in beauty therapy			

	Short wave length	Long wave length
Cosmic		0.002 nm
Gamma	0.002 nm	0.14 nm
X-rays	0.14 nm	13.4 nm
Ultraviolet	10 nm	400 nm
Visible	400 nm	770 nm
Infrared	770 nm	400,000 nm
Radio	100,000 nm	

Frequency

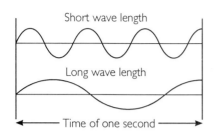

Figure 7.3 *Rays of different wave lengths will have different frequencies*

The bands of the spectrum also have different frequencies. Frequency is the number of complete waves that pass a point in one second. Many more waves of short wave length will pass the point in one second than those of long wave length.

The rays of shorter wave length will have a higher frequency than the rays of longer wave length. In other words, as the wave length increases the frequency decreases. (The term frequency is familiar to us when tuning the radio; programmes are transmitted on the radio at different frequencies)

UNITS OF FREQUENCIES

Frequency is measured in hertz (Hz). The number of waves past a point in one second is the number of hertz, eg 50 waves passing a point per second = 50 Hz. For higher frequencies the units become

1 kilohertz (kHz)	= 1,000 Hz
1 megahertz (mHz)	= 1,000 kHz

Properties and laws of radiation

In order to give the most effective and safe treatment, the beauty therapist should be aware of certain laws and principles which govern the behaviour of rays/waves. Both infrared, visible light and ultraviolet rays will travel in straight lines until they meet a new medium, where they may be refracted, reflected or absorbed.

REFRACTION

This is the bending of rays when they meet a new medium; a common example is looking at a stick held in water – it appears to bend. Refraction occurs when rays pass from one medium to another, eg from air through glass or water. The rays striking the part are known as incident rays, or the ray of incidence. If the incident rays strike the part at right angles, they will pass straight through. If the rays strike the part at an angle, they will bend towards or away from the *normal* depending on the medium. (The *normal* is an imaginary line which lies perpendicular to the surface.)

● If the rays pass into a more dense medium, they will bend towards the normal.

● If they pass into a less dense medium, they will bend away from
the normal.

Figure 7.4   *Refraction*

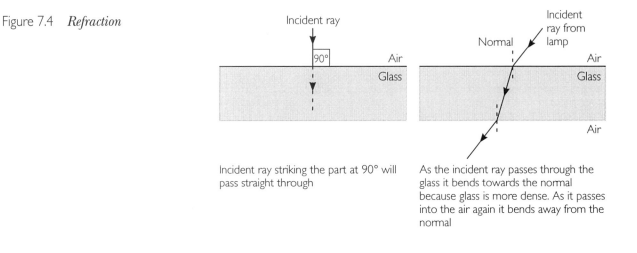

Incident ray striking the part at 90° will
pass straight through

As the incident ray passes through the
glass it bends towards the normal
because glass is more dense. As it passes
into the air again it bends away from the
normal

REFLECTION

This is the reflection of rays when they meet a surface. Shiny or
white surfaces reflect more rays than dark surfaces, which absorb
rays, eg a greater proportion of light rays will be reflected by snow
than by soil. A mirror is designed to reflect rays.

The law of reflection states that the angle of incidence is equal to
the angle of reflection. To measure these angles, an imaginary line
is drawn perpendicular to the surface struck by the rays, this is the
normal.

● The angle of incidence lies between the ray of incidence and
the normal.

● The angle of reflection lies between the ray of reflection and
the normal.

Figure 7.5   *Reflection*

The normal is an imaginary line at right
angles (90°) to the surface

x is the angle of incidence
y is the angle of reflection.
These are always equal

X is the angle of incidence.
Y is the angle of reflection.
These are always equal.

The angle of incidence is one of the factors governing the proportion of rays absorbed by the medium which the rays strike. This is an important consideration when giving UV and IR treatments, as the effectiveness of the treatments will depend on the number of rays absorbed.

ABSORPTION

The law of Grotthus states that: 'rays must be absorbed to produce an effect'.

The amount of absorption and consequently the effect depends on the following:

1 The wave length and frequency of the rays:
   (a) Infrared is absorbed at a level of 3 mm approximately.
   (b) Ultraviolet is absorbed at a level of 1 mm approximately. (This is dealt with in greater depth on page 148.)
2 The type of medium:
   (a) Certain substances absorb rays while others allow the rays to pass through, eg window glass absorbs most ultraviolet rays but allows visible rays to pass through.
   (b) Sun glasses are especially designed to absorb ultraviolet rays but allow visible rays to pass through. In the same way, body tissues absorb certain wave lengths at certain levels, but allow others to pass through.
3 The angle at which the rays strike the part also affects absorption. The cosine law governs the way intensity hence absorption is affected by the angle of incidence.

THE COSINE LAW

This law states that the intensity of radiation at a surface varies with the cosine of the angle of incidence (ie the angle between the incident ray and the normal).

Figure 7.6   *Cosine law*

Incident ray striking the surface at 90°.
There is no reflection, therefore there is maximum absorption

If the incident rays strike the part at 90 degrees, there will be no angle between the incident ray and the normal (it is 0 degrees);

here there is maximum intensity and absorption. As the incident ray moves down towards the surface, the angle increases and the intensity decreases.

Figure 7.7   *Incident ray striking at different angles*

Incident ray striking the part at different angles

X and Y are the angles of incidence.

As the angle becomes greater X to Y, the intensity at the surface decreases. The amount of decrease can be calculated by measuring the angle between the incident ray and the normal and looking up its cosine in the cosine tables.

The cosine of 0° is 1
The cosine of 60° is 0.5

Therefore, if the angle of incidence moves from 0 degrees to 60 degrees, the intensity is halved. It will diminish further as the angle increases. In order to ensure the most effective treatment, the rays must strike the part at 90 degrees; this will ensure maximum intensity, absorption and effect, eg the sun's rays are more likely to burn at midday when the sun is at right angles than in the late afternoon, when it is low in the sky (if the exposure time is the same).

Intensity of radiation

The intensity of radiation will depend on three factors:

1 The intensity of the lamp.
2 The distance between the lamp and the skin.
3 The angle at which the rays strike the part.

THE INTENSITY OF THE LAMP

Lamps vary in output and, therefore, intensity; some have control dials for increasing and decreasing intensity. The intensity from infrared lamps does not pose any problems, as the client is able to feel if the intensity is too high and the distance can be increased or lamp turned down. However, ultraviolet rays do not give out heat and cannot be felt; therefore, the distance and time of exposure must be carefully calculated to produce the required effect. This is calculated using the patch test. The patch test procedure is only relevant when using mercury vapour lamps for treating conditions such as acne. It is not necessary to carry out this test when giving sunbed treatments.

Sunbeds are designed to emit certain intensities at their set distance and so produce the required effect in a certain time. Manufacturer's instructions should be adhered to and consideration given to sensitivity of the client, eg skin type and previous exposure. (This is discussed fully on page 161.)

THE DISTANCE BETWEEN THE LAMP AND THE SKIN

The law of inverse squares governs intensity in relation to distance. The law of inverse squares states that the intensity from a point source (ie the lamp) varies inversely with the square of the distance from the point source. In other words, the intensity varies inversely with the square of the distance from the source.

- If the distance increases, the intensity decreases by the square of the distance.
- If the distance decreases, the intensity increases by the square of the distance.
- If you double the distance the intensity is quartered.
- If you reduce the distance by half, the intensity will increase four times (quadrupled).

Figure 7.8 *Radiation from a point source illustrating the law of inverse squares*

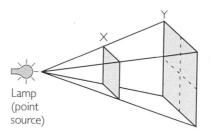

X is one meter from the source.
Y is two meters from the source.

If the client is placed at distance X, she will receive the calculated dose. If the distance is increased to Y (ie doubled), then the intensity is a quarter of that at X.

To produce the same effect on the skin when changing distances of UV lamps the following apply:

- If you halve the distance, you quarter the time.
- If you double the distance, you quadruple the time.

THE ANGLE AT WHICH THE RAYS STRIKE THE PART

The cosine law governs intensity in relation to the angle of incidence. This is fully discussed on page 137.

When giving radiation treatments, ie infrared or ultraviolet, the lamp should be positioned so that the rays strike the part at 90 degrees. This will ensure maximum intensity, absorption and effect.

Note never position lamps directly over the client; the client should be positioned and the lamp angled so that the rays can strike at 90 degrees.

Infrared rays

Figure 7.9   *An infrared lamp*

Infrared rays are electromagnetic waves with wave lengths between 700 nm and 400,000 nm. They are given off from the sun and any hot object, eg electric fires, gas and coal fires, hot packs and various types of lamps.

The lamps that produce infrared rays can be divided into two main types:

1 The non-luminous type (called the infrared lamps).
2 The luminous type (called radiant heat lamps).

Both these types of lamp emit infrared rays. The difference lies in their wave length. The non-luminous type emit rays of longer wave length, around 4,000 nm, while the luminous type emit rays of shorter wave, around 1,000 nm and include waves from the visible spectrum and UVL. The differing wave lengths produce slightly different effects when absorbed by body tissues.

THE NON-LUMINOUS LAMPS

Many types of non-luminous lamps are produced, but they all have a non-glowing source that emits infrared rays. A common type uses a coil of wire embedded in fire clay, which is placed in the centre of a reflector. When the lamp is switched on, the wire gets hot and heats the fire clay; the rays are then emitted from the hot fire clay, they pass through the air and are absorbed by a body placed in their path. The rays from non-luminous lamps are of longer wave length, are invisible, are less irritating and less penetrating than the short rays from luminous lamps. They may feel hotter at equal distances and power due to increased absorption in the top layers of the skin. These wave lengths are further from visible light and are consequently called *far IR*.

THE LUMINOUS LAMPS (RADIANT HEAT LAMPS)

These lamps give off infrared rays from glowing or incandescent sources, such as hot wires or powerful bulbs. These are also placed in the centre of a reflector. When the lamp is switched on, the wire glows, giving off infrared and visible rays and small amounts of ultraviolet rays. Some bulbs have filters to cut out some visible rays and ultraviolet rays, these bulbs are usually red in colour.

The rays produced by these lamps have a shorter wave length, include some visible rays, are more penetrating (down to the subcutaneous layer) and are more irritating than the rays from non-luminous lamps. These wave lengths are nearer visible light and are consequently called *near IR*.

Table H *Comparisons of luminous and non-luminous lamps*

Non-luminous	Luminous
Long wave length around 4,000 nm	Shorter wave length around 1,000 nm
Include no visible rays	Include some visible rays and a small amount of UVL.
Penetrates approximately 1 mm of skin	Penetrates approximately 3 mm of tissue
Less irritating	More irritating
May feel hotter at equal power and distance	Will feel less hot at equal power and distance
Takes 10–15 minutes to heat up	Heats up quickly, approximately 2 minutes

COMBINED INFRARED AND ULTRAVIOLET LAMPS

Ultraviolet rays are part of the electromagnetic spectrum with a shorter wave length than infrared rays and visible light rays from 400 nm to 10 nm. These UVL rays are not used for heating effects, but for other effects, such as tanning etc (see page 155).

Figure 7.10   *A combined infrared and ultraviolet lamp*

Some lamps are manufactured with two elements, one producing UVL rays and the other producing infrared rays. These lamps can be dangerous in inexperienced or incompetent hands. Therapists who do not distinguish between the two may give long duration of UVL, by pressing the wrong switch.

- UVL glows giving a blue/white colour.
- IR gives invisible rays or glows red/orange.

Manufacturers produce a wide variety of lamps, tunnels, solariums (combined UV), and the therapist should familiarise herself with all the lamps she finds in her salon.

- Examine all lamps carefully and read manufacturer's instructions.
- Check stability.
- Check joints and screws for angling the lamp; are they tight and secure?
- How can the angle of the lamp be changed?
- Is there an on/off switch on the lamp, or must it be switched on/off at the wall socket?
- Is there an intensity control, or must intensity be controlled by increasing or decreasing the distance?
- Is it in good order; check the plugs, reflector, grid etc.
- Is it dual purpose, ie infrared and ultraviolet light; if so make sure which switch operates infrared and which for ultraviolet.

Infrared irradiation of the body

Infrared is used by the beauty therapist to heat body tissues. It may be used to treat localised areas or the body in general.

USES

1 As a general heating treatment to promote relaxation.
2 As a localised treatment for relief of pain and tension.
3 In facial work to aid the absorption of certain products.
4 As a pre-heating treatment, either generally or locally, to increase the circulation and thus make following treatments more effective.

EFFECTS OF INFRARED RADIATION

HEATING OF BODY TISSUES

When infrared rays are absorbed by the tissues, heat is produced in the area. The rays from luminous generators penetrate more deeply than those from non-luminous lamps, therefore, superficial and deeper tissues are heated directly. With non-luminous lamps the top 1 mm of skin is heated directly, but the deeper tissues are heated by conduction.

INCREASED METABOLIC RATE

(Van't Hoffs law states that a chemical reaction capable of being accelerated will be accelerated by heat.)

Metabolism is a chemical change which will be accelerated by heat. The increase in metabolic rate will be greatest where the heating is greatest, ie in the superficial tissues; therefore more oxygen and nutrients are required and more waste products and metabolites are produced.

VASODILATION WITH INCREASE IN CIRCULATION

Heat has a direct effect on the blood vessels producing vasodilation and an increase in blood flow in an attempt to cool the area. Vasodilation is also produced by stimulation of sensory nerve endings which cause reflex dilation of arterioles.

Vasodilation is also produced as a result of the increase in metabolic rate and increase in waste products. The metabolites act on the walls of capillaries and arterioles causing dilation.

The heat-regulating centre of the brain will be stimulated as body heat rises. This will result in general dilation of superficial vessels to ensure that the body is not overheated. Hyperaemia is the term used to describe an increase in the flow of blood to the area due to vasodilation. Erythema means reddening of the skin due to hyperaemia and vasodilation.

FALL IN BLOOD PRESSURE

If the superficial blood vessels dilate, the peripheral resistance is reduced and this will result in a fall in blood pressure. (When blood flows through vessels with small lumen, it exerts a certain pressure on the walls. If the lumen is increased by the vessels dilating, the pressure on the walls will be reduced.)

Figure 7.11   *Pressure on vessel walls*

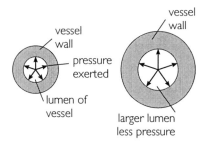

INCREASE IN HEART RATE

The increased metabolism and circulation means that the heart must beat faster to meet the demand; therefore, the heart rate increases.

GENERAL RISE IN BODY TEMPERATURE

When one area of the body is heated for a prolonged time, there is a general rise in body temperature by conduction and convection. The heat will spread through surrounding tissues and will be carried by the blood circulating through the area.

INCREASED ACTIVITY OF SWEAT GLANDS

As the body temperature rises, the heat regulating centres in the brain are affected. The sweat glands are then stimulated to produce more sweat in order to lose body heat. This increases the elimination of waste products.

EFFECTS ON MUSCLE TISSUE

Muscle tissue is affected in two ways:

1 The rise in temperature produces muscle relaxation and relieves tension and pain.

2 The increase in circulation provides the nutrients and oxygen necessary for muscle action and the removal of waste is speeded up.

When muscles are warm, they contract more efficiently than when they are cold.

EFFECTS ON SENSORY NERVES

Heat has a soothing effect on sensory nerve endings. However, intense heat has an irritating effect.

PIGMENTATION

Repeated and intense exposure to infrared produces a purple or brown mottled appearance on the area. This may be due to destruction of blood cells and release of haemoglobin.

CONTRA-INDICATIONS

1 Areas of defective skin sensation and hypersensitive skin.
2 Heart conditions and blood pressure disorders (high or low).
3 Thrombosis or phlebitis or any areas of deficient circulation.
4 Heavy colds and fevers.
5 Migraines and headaches.
6 Skin disorders and diseases.
7 Diabetes, as skin sensitivity may be impaired.
8 Recent scar tissue (defective sensitivity).
9 Extensive bruising.
10 Recent exposure to UVL (sunburn).
11 Body infrared would not be given in the last four months of pregnancy or first two days of a heavy period.
12 Any area where liniments or ointments have been applied.

DANGERS

1 Burns may be caused
  (a) if the heat is too intense;
  (b) if the client is too near the lamp and fails to report overheating;
  (c) if the skin sensation is defective and the client may not be aware of overheating;
  (d) if the client touches the lamp;

(e) if the lamp should fall and touch the client, or the bedding; overheating of pillows and blankets can cause fire and burns.

2 Electric shock from faulty apparatus or water on the treatment area producing a short circuit.

3 Headache: irradiating the back of the neck and head or over heating by prolonged exposure may cause headache.

4 Faintness: overheating or extensive irradiation may cause a fall in blood pressure, which may cause faintness.

5 Damage to the eyes: infrared exposure of the eyes can cause cataracts; a client should close her eyes and turn away from the lamp, wear goggles or have cotton wool over her eyes.

6 Constipation: this may occur following prolonged exposure and if water loss through sweating is not replaced by water intake.

7 Chill: this may occur if the client goes out into the cold too quickly after exposure.

PRECAUTIONS

1 Clean the skin with cologne to remove sebum.

2 Ensure a safe distance of the lamp from the client. This distance depends on the client's tolerance and the output of the lamp (18–36 inch, 45–90 cm).

3 Do not place the lamp directly over the client.

4 Ensure that the lamp is stable with the head over a foot if lamp has three or five feet.

5 Ensure that the lamp is in good working order and that there are no dents in the reflector.

6 Ensure that the flexes are sound and not trailing in a walking area.

7 Check for contra-indications.

8 Carry out a hot and cold sensitivity test (see below).

9 Protect the eyes.

10 Explain the importance of calling immediately if the client feels too hot.

11 Warn the client not to move nearer to or touch the lamp.

TREATMENT TECHNIQUE

PREPARATION OF THE CLIENT

1 Place the client in a comfortable position (when treating areas of the back, use side lying or the recovery position, well supported by pillows. If treating knees, use half lying).

2 Check that all jewellery has been removed.

3 Clean the area with cologne to remove sebum.

4 Check for contra-indications.

5 Explain the treatment to the client.

6 Carry out a sensitivity test using two test tubes one filled with hot water the other with cold water. Instruct the client to close her eyes. Carry out the test all over the area to be irradiated. Touch the client with either the hot test tube or the cold test tube at random over the area. Ask her if she feels hot or cold. (If the client cannot tell the difference between hot and cold, she has defective sensation and the treatment should not be carried out.)

7 Cover the areas not receiving treatment.

8 Warn the client that warmth should be comfortable and to call if the heat becomes too intense.

9 Warn the client not to touch lamp or move closer to it.

Figure 7.12   *Positioning of the lamp*

PROCEDURE

1 Check the plug, leads and reflector.

2 Switch the lamp on directed towards floor.

(a) IR takes 10–15 minutes to reach maximum output.

(b) Radiant heat (visible) takes around 2 minutes.

3 When maximum intensity is reached, position the lamp ensuring stability. (If the lamp has three feet, place the head of the lamp over one of the feet, ensuring that the angle joints are secure).

4 Make sure that the face of the lamp is parallel with the part so that the *rays strike the part at 90 degrees* for maximum penetration, absorption and effect. Do not place the lamp directly above the client. (This also applies if infrared rays are being used as a pre-heating treatment.)

5 Select an appropriate distance between 45–90 cms (18–36 in). The selected distance depends on two factors:

(a) the intensity of the lamp;

(b) the client's tolerance.

(60 cm (24 in) is a good average.)

6 Ensure that the rays are not irradiating the client's face. (The lamp should not be irradiating the eyes or face of the client nor the therapist). If using infrared rays for facial work, the eyes must be closed and covered with cotton wool.

7 Observe the client throughout the treatment.

8 Treatment time is 20–30 minutes, until the desired effect is obtained.

9 The treatment may be followed by massage or electrical treatments, but not UVL. (Infrared given before ultraviolet increases the sensitivity of the client and intensifies the reaction with risk of overdose.) Infrared may be used after overexposure to UVL to reduce the reaction. The client should not rise suddenly after infrared treatment (as the blood pressure is lowered and she may feel faint.)

POINTS TO CONSIDER WHEN POSITIONING THE LAMP

1 Ensure a safe but effective distance from the part.

2 Never place the lamp directly over the client. If it falls or the bulb breaks, it would cause burns to client.

3 Position the lamp so that the surface of the lamp is parallel with the part and the rays strike the part at 90 degrees for maximum penetration, absorption and effect. This applies whenever the lamp is used.

4 Avoid the face and eyes.

Ultraviolet radiation

Ultraviolet rays are part of the electromagnetic spectrum with wave lengths of between 400 nm and 10 nm, they lie between the violet end of the visible spectrum and X-rays. Ultraviolet rays are divided into three bands according to their wave length:

- UVA with the longest wave length – 315–400 nm
- UVB the middle band with wave length – 280–315 nm
- UVC the shortest wave length – below 280 nm

The wave length determines the penetration and effects of the rays. The skin acts as a protective layer, which absorbs ultraviolet rays, preventing damage of deeper tissues.

- UVA penetrates down to the capillary loops in the dermis. This causes tanning and damage to the skin's connective tissue i.e. the elastin and collagen fibres. It may increase the risk of skin cancer.

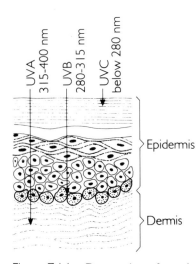

Figure 7.14   *Penetration of rays into the skin*

- UVB penetrates as far as the lower levels of the epidermis – the stratum basale. This causes tanning and also sunburn. Over exposure will cause skin cancer.
- UVC penetrates only the upper layer of the epidermis – the stratum corneum. This will damage skin cells, and destroy bacteria (abiotic).

SOURCES OF ULTRAVIOLET RADIATION

1 Natural sunlight emits all ultraviolet rays. The intensity of UV reaching the earth's surface will vary with the time of year, the time of day, with altitude, latitude and variations in cloud cover and shade. The intensity of radiation will also increase with reflection from light surfaces, such as snow and rippling water. The destructive and harmful UVC rays are absorbed and screened out as they travel through the atmosphere; they do not reach the earth's surface. The effects of natural sunlight are therefore due to UVA and UVB. There is growing concern that as the ozone layer is becoming thinner and holes are developing; the harmful UVC rays will reach the earth.

2 Artificial sunlight is produced by high or low pressure tubes and lamps. In hospital departments, sun lamps are used to treat a wide variety of medical conditions. These emit UVA, UVB and some UVC rays. In the salon, sunbeds and solariums are used for tanning the body. All the harmful UVC rays and most, if not all, of the burning UVB rays are filtered out of these beds. However, there are dangers associated with their use and operators who use them should be made aware of these.

THE HIGH PRESSURE MERCURY VAPOUR LAMPS

This lamp has a U-shaped or straight burner made of quartz. This is placed in the centre of a parabolic reflector (quartz is used as it allows all ultraviolet rays to pass through whereas glass does not). The tube contains argon gas and a small quantity of mercury. An electrode is sealed in at either end of the tube. When the current is switched on, the argon ionises and electrons flow through the tube. The mercury vaporises and ionises giving off ultraviolet light. This type of lamp emits UVA, UVB, some UVC, visible and infrared rays.

These lamps with U-shaped burners are mainly found in hospital departments for the treatment of acne, alopecia, psoriasis, etc. Although the small amount of the shortest destructive UVC rays are absorbed by the air, the UVB can cause burning. Great care has to be taken when using these lamps. A patch test is always carried out at the commencement of treatment to determine the skin reaction to the lamp, (see page 165).

- The distance between the lamp and client must be carefully measured and recorded. The time of exposure must also be recorded.
- The progression of each dose must be calculated.
- The total running time of the lamp must be recorded, as with use the tube becomes more opaque and the intensity is diminished.
- Although these lamps are not usually found in the beauty salon, the therapist should be aware of the necessary precautions if asked to use one.

Figure 7.15   *A mercury vapour lamp*

THE OVERHEAD SOLARIUM

These are usually suspended at a fixed distance above the bed. They contain elements producing infrared rays and tubes producing ultraviolet rays. They are very relaxing for the client, giving off a mild warmth and producing a tan. They emit infrared rays, visible light, UVA, and some UVB; filters are used to control the ultraviolet emission and cut out unwanted UVB rays and all UVC rays.

There is usually an alarm clock which is set to ring halfway through the treatment to indicate that the client should turn over, and an automatic switch off at the end of the treatment. There are slight variations in the solariums available and manufacturers' instructions should be carefully studied and adhered to. Particular care must be taken with pale, sensitive-skinned clients. Worn out bulbs, tubes and filters must be replaced by the exact same models provided by the manufacturers.

SUNBEDS

These come in various forms to irradiate one side of the body or both sides simultaneously. More modern beds are slightly curved to irradiate the sides of the body as well as front and back. The beds are made up of a collection of fluorescent tubes closely packed together. The tubes are around 120 cm in length and made of vita glass, which is coated on the inside with a phosphorus lining. This lining is designed to absorb UVC rays and most if not all UVB rays. The tubes contain argon gas and some mercury with electrodes sealed at either end. When the current is switched on, the argon ionises and electrons flow through the tube. The mercury ionises and vaporises and UVL is emitted. The phosphorus coating absorbs unwanted harmful rays. Some beds emit only UVA and tan slowly while others emit mainly UVA (96–98 per cent) and a small amount of UVB (2–4 per cent). These beds tan more quickly and the tan lasts longer.

The tubes are packed together side by side. There may be reflectors behind the tubes or tubes may have inbuilt reflectors so that more tubes can be incorporated into the bed giving a higher intensity of radiation.

The distance between the tubes and the surface to be irradiated is fixed and the beds are designed to produce a certain effect in a set time. The time of exposure will vary depending on the sensitivity of the client. The therapist should never assume that one sunbed is the same as another, exposure times may be different and will depend on the intensity of the radiation and skin type; manufacturer's instructions must be carefully studied and followed.

There are certain features common to all beds. They have an on/off switch and timer control; some have an emergency button for quick release. This should always be explained to the client and she should be able to reach the switches from the exposure position. The more modern sunbeds have a fan to control the heating.

- A sunbed should always be positioned in a well-ventilated room to prevent build up of ozone which is damaging to the respiratory system and also to dissipate the heat generated by the sunbed.
- It should be isolated in its own room or behind a full-length partition so that all rays are contained and cannot irradiate other clients.
- The bed should be wiped over before and after treatment with a disinfecting detergent. Appropriate detergents supplied by the

sunbed manufacturer must be used, as other detergents may damage or form a film on the acrylic surfaces, they may be toxic or inflammable, or could possibly sensitise the skin of the client.

- Sunbeds require little maintenance, but they should be regularly inspected for electrical and mechanical safety, and any faulty or exhausted tubes replaced immediately, with identical tubes supplied by the manufacturer. Servicing and repair should be carried out by a qualified electrician in accordance with information supplied by the manufacturer.

- The running time of the sunbed must be recorded as the tubes wear out with use and the intensity is reduced. Always check the manufacturer's instructions as the working life of tubes will vary from sunbed to sunbed. The intensity of some tubes is reduced by half after 500 hours, while others are exhausted.

- Always replace tubes with the exact same model as the power of tubes will vary; they must be replaced by tubes of equal power and design in order to maintain radiation output. This also applies to filters.

USES OF ULTRAVIOLET RADIATION

1 *Tanning (dose E1–E2)*. This is the most common use in the beauty salon. It enhances appearance and gives a feeling of well-being.
2 *Tonic effect (dose E1)*. UVL is thought to have a general tonic effect. Improving appetite and sleep while reducing irritability and nervousness.
3 *Treatment of acne (dose E2)*.
   (a) The increase in circulation will improve the condition of the skin.
   (b) Ultraviolet has a drying effect on the skin, reducing sebum.
   (c) Desquamation following exposure will aid removal of comedones and relieve blockages.
   (d) Ultraviolet has an abiotic effect on the skin.

In hospitals, UVL is used in the treatment of: wounds and ulcers, psoriasis, alopecia areata and totalis, and to produce vitamin D in the treatment and prevention of rickets.

EXPOSURE TO NATURAL SUNLIGHT

THE EFFECTS OF EXPOSURE TO NATURAL SUNLIGHT

The effects of UV radiation on the skin will depend on the intensity of radiation and on the skin type. Dermatologists list six skin types which will react differently to the same exposure:

Type 1: never tans, always burns.
Type 2: tans with difficulty, burns frequently.
Type 3: tans easily, burns rarely.
Type 4: always tans, never burns.
Type 5: genetically brown skin (Asian or Mongoloid).
Type 6: genetically black skin (Negroid).

Everyone is familiar with the acute effect of over-exposure to natural sunlight, namely, sunburn. There is erythema with swelling, sometimes blistering followed by extensive peeling and itching. The chronic effects of regular exposure are dryness of the skin, wrinkles, laxity and variations in skin pigmentation, which may show freckling, vitiligo or chloasma.

Some individuals react abnormally to sunlight and develop a variety of conditions and eruptions, known as polymorphic light eruptions. The skin becomes red and oedematous with itchy, hard papules or scaling.

Certain drugs and cosmetics increase the risk of photosensitivity reaction; this may be an itchy, painful rash followed by pronounced, sometimes permanent, pigmentation. The most serious effect of over- or prolonged exposure to sunlight is the risk of inducing skin cancer. There is considerable evidence to suggest that prolonged exposure to natural sunlight, ie UVA and UVB rays will cause degenerative skin changes and carcinomas. Those in the high-risk category are: outdoor workers, such as farmers and fishermen; fair, pale-skinned types 1 and 2, especially those living in areas of high intensity sunlight, such as Australia and near the Equator; individuals whose skins are not normally exposed to sunlight, but occasionally receive short-term intense exposure are also at risk.

In addition to causing skin damage, ultraviolet radiation is also damaging to the cornea and lens of the eye. Polarising lenses should always be worn to protect the eye in sunlight.

There is increasing evidence that prolonged radiation will impair the function of the immune system by causing disturbances and reductions in the numbers of lymphocytes. There is a growing awareness of these hazards among the general public, but the beauty therapist has a role to play in educating and giving advice to clients. Clients should be made aware of the following precautions to be taken in natural sunlight:

I Individuals with fair or red hair, blue eyes and sensitive, pale skin who tan rarely and burn easily should take particular care. They should avoid exposure to strong sunlight.

2 Prolonged exposure to sunlight, whether occupational or recreational, should be avoided, and so should infrequent short bursts of intensive exposure.

3 Sunscreens with a sun protection factor (SPF) of at least 6 should be used. The higher the number, the greater the protection. This sunscreen should be applied before exposure and renewed every two hours and after swimming.

4 Lengthy exposure should be avoided particularly, between 11 am and 4 pm, when the sun is at its highest. Begin with a short exposure of 10–30 minutes on the first day and increase gradually each day. At other times, wear long-sleeved clothing and a hat and find some shade.

5 Avoid sunbathing if taking drugs (see page 160).

6 Remember that UV rays will pass through light cloud; it is, therefore, possible to burn on a cloudy day or on a sunny, windy day although it may feel cool.

THE USE OF ARTIFICIAL SUNLIGHT FOR TANNING

Sunbeds and solariums are used for tanning the body. Some sunbeds emit UVA and a small percentage of UVB, while others have been developed to emit UVA only in the belief that they will produce a tan without any harmful effects. Dermatologists dispute this claim and the British Photodermatology Group have gathered strong evidence to show that prolonged exposure to UVA is harmful. They recommend that the use of sunbeds for tanning should be discouraged. They admit that more research is required and that there are gaps in knowledge. Exposure to UVA may produce effects similar to natural sunlight. Some individuals may develop erythema, burning sensation, itching (pruritis), dryness, freckling, polymorphic light eruption, photo sensitisation, impairment of immune function and damage of the lens and cornea of the eye. Prolonged UVA exposure may cause degenerative skin changes and may accelerate the development of certain skin cancers (to date this has only been proven in mice exposed to UVA).

Manufacturers state that there is insufficient evidence to support these claims. The decision to use a sunbed is a matter of personal choice and, despite the evidence, the use of sunbeds is extremely popular. The British Photodermatology Group have issued guidelines for those who operate and use sunbeds:

1 The use of sunbeds should not exceed two courses per year.

2 No more than ten sessions per course.

3 Each session should be timed to produce a barely perceptible erythema 8–24 hours later, and should not exceed 30 minutes per session. (This limits exposure to 10 hours per year.)

Several groups should never use sunbeds:

1 Children under 16 years.
2 People who burn easily.
3 People who do not tan or tan poorly – types 1 and 2.
4 Those taking drugs or using cosmetics which cause photosensitivity.
5 Those suffering from skin disorders aggravated by sunlight.
6 Those with a history of skin cancer.
7 Those with risk factors for cutaneous melanoma, eg multiple naevii, overdose in the past.

GENERAL EFFECTS OF EXPOSURE TO ARTIFICIAL SUNLIGHT

ERYTHEMA

Erythema reaction following ultraviolet irradiation differs from the erythema reaction following infrared irradiation in that it does not appear immediately. It takes 6–12 hours for the redness to appear, and occurs due to the irritation of cells of the epidermis. The ultraviolet rays that reach the lower levels of the epidermis, ie UVA and UVB, damage and destroy some of the cells. This results in the chemical histamine being released in response to the injury. The histamine causes the blood vessels to dilate, bringing an increase in blood flow and thus producing an erythema.

Further irritation will cause greater dilation and an exudation of fluid from the vessels into the tissue spaces forming blisters. Sensory nerves will be stimulated giving soreness and pain.

The greater the ultraviolet dose, the greater the irritation, therefore, the more histamine will be released and the greater will be the erythema reaction. It takes some time for these processes to occur, hence the 6–12 hours before reaction appears.

There are four degrees of erythema:

1st degree (E1): slight reddening, no irritation, no pigmentation, fades in 24 hours, no desquamation.
2nd degree (E2): deeper reddening, slight irritation, slight pigmentation, fades 2–3 days, powdery desquamation.
3rd degree (E3): skin is very red, hot, sore and oedematous, itchy, marked pigmentation, fades 7–10 days, sheets of skin lift off.
4th degree (E4): similar to E3 but blisters form, may be necessary to receive hospital treatment.

TANNING

Tanning develops within two days of radiation. It is produced by the action of UVA and UVB on the melanocytes in the skin. Melanocytes are specialised cells found in the basal layer or stratum germinativum of the epidermis. These branching cells produce the pigment melanin and extend upwards to provide a protective cover over the living nucleated cells of the epidermis. As the pigmentation is built up, the penetration of the rays is reduced and destruction and damage of cells lessened. Melanin is formed by the action of UVA and UVB on the amino acid *tyrosine*. Two types of melanin are produced *eumelanin*, which produces a dark brown or black colour, and *phaeomelanin*, which produces a yellowish to red colour. The variation of brown colour found in different skin types depends upon the percentages eumelanin and phaeomelanin produced.

Tanning of the skin is produced in two ways:

1 *Immediate tanning or quick tanning*. This is produced by the UVA rays wave length 400–315 nm. These rays stimulate and darken the melanin granules already in the skin. It requires long exposure to UVA and fades quickly within a few days. UVA will produce a tan in those individuals who tan easily (Type 3). Type 1 and 2 or areas without a previous tan may not tan.

2 *Delayed tanning*. This requires a high dose of UVA, but is produced by a low dose of UVB. These rays stimulate the melanocytes to produce new dark melanin granules. Once started, this process will continue and will produce a longer lasting tan. Therefore the most effective tanning is produced by sunbeds emitting UVA and a very low percentage of UVB. The tanning response to ultraviolet depends on the skin (see page 161). Sensitive skins burn easily but tan very slowly; some very sensitive skins will not tan at all. Types 1 and 2 should avoid using sunbeds or keep to very low exposure times of 10 minutes for the first dose and increasing by 5 minutes each session. If there is any sign of burning, further exposure should be avoided until the erythema has completely died down.

Type 3 skins of medium sensitivity burn less easily and tan more quickly. They can take a longer exposure time without burning around 15–20 minutes for the first exposure. Dark olive skins tan quickly and rarely burn and can take longer exposure times.

THICKENING OF THE EPIDERMIS

The UVB radiation penetrates down to the stratum basale or stratum germinativum. The irritation caused to these cells produces over activity and increased mitosis. These rapidly multiplying cells push upwards and form a marked thickening of the stratum corneum. This may become three times its normal thickness. This acts as a protection to reduce ultraviolet penetration. The dosage must, therefore, be increased with each exposure to produce the same effect, unless extensive peeling has occurred.

When using UVL for therapeutic purposes, it is sometimes necessary to maintain preset erythema doses and the length of exposure must be increased each time to produce the same effect. In order to maintain an:

E1 the timing must be increased by 25 per cent.
E2 the timing must be increased by 50 per cent.

This does not apply when using sunbeds for tanning purposes.

SKIN PEELING (DESQUAMATION)

The normal process of desquamation is accelerated due to an increase in mitotic activity of the stratum basale and migration of cells to the surface. The amount of peeling depends on the intensity of exposure and the erythema reaction.

1st degree erythema, peeling hardly noticeable.
2nd degree erythema, fine powdery flaking.
3rd and 4th degree erythema, marked peeling with large flakes or sheets.

Peeling reduces the protection gained by the thickened epidermis.

PRODUCTION OF VITAMIN D

Ultraviolet radiation of the skin causes a chemical reaction which converts 7-dehydro-cholesterol found in sebum into cholecalciferol, namely, vitamin D_3.

Vitamin D is necessary for the absorption of calcium and phosphorus, which play a part in the formation and growth of teeth and bones (lack of vitamin D causes rickets). Calcium is also an important factor in the blood clotting mechanism. This production of vitamin D is important beneficial effect of ultraviolet light on the skin.

GENERAL TONIC EFFECT

General ultraviolet irradiation has a tonic effect on the body. Appetite and sleep are improved; irritability and nervousness may be reduced.

ABIOTIC EFFECT

The rays of short wave length UVC rays are abiotic rays as they destroy bacteria and micro-organisms. They are used in germicidal lamps or cabinets. These rays can be used to destroy and prevent the growth of bacteria in wounds. UVC rays are absorbed as they pass through air; therefore, they would not reach the skin from lamps placed some distance away. Special lamps called kromeyer lamps have to be used. These have enclosed tubes that are water cooled to prevent heating. They can be used in close contact with the wounds and are used in hospitals to promote healing. They are not found in beauty salons.

SKIN AGEING (SOLAR ELASTOSIS OR PHOTOAGEING)

As previously mentioned, when ultraviolet rays penetrate the skin they damage cells. UVB will damage cells down to the basal layer, as this is the limit of their penetration. UVA rays penetrate into the dermis and damage dermal cells and fibres (ie the elastin and collagen fibres). This produces loss of elasticity, laxity and wrinkling of the skin. Damage of cells will eventually produce thinning and dryness of the skin. Increased over activity of some melanocytes will produce freckling and liver spots, while absence of melanocytes in other areas leave white, unpigmented patches. All these factors contribute to premature ageing of the skin. Prolonged exposure to all ultraviolet radiation should be avoided.

CARCINOGENIC EFFECT

There are three main types of skin cancer:

1 basal cell carcinoma;
2 squamous cell carcinoma;
3 malignant melanoma.

There is increasing evidence to link prolonged exposure to natural sunlight, ie UVA and UVB, with skin degeneration and skin cancer. It was thought that only UVB rays were responsible, but it is now thought UVA rays may also have a carcinogenic effect. To date, the development of squamous cell carcinoma has been reported in mice exposed to UVA, but it has yet to be proven that UVA exposure alone induces carcinoma in humans.

The ultraviolet rays penetrating the skin affect the DNA in the nucleus of the cells. This interferes with the replication of the cells predisposing to skin cancer. Fair or pale skinned individuals who burn easily and tan rarely (types 1 and 2) are vulnerable as are those with multiple naevi or with previous history of severe sunburn. Long exposures to natural sunlight and prolonged frequent use of sunbeds should be avoided.

DAMAGING EFFECT ON THE EYES

The tough outer coating of the eye called the cornea and the lens of the eye can be adversely affected by radiation. UVB and UVC rays are absorbed by the cornea and do not penetrate further. High intensity exposure to these shorter wave lengths may induce keratitis (inflammation of the cornea) and conjunctivitis (inflammation of the conjunctiva). Both these conditions are extremely irritating and painful.

The long UVA rays penetrate further and are absorbed by the lens; over exposure can cause opaqueness of the lens known as cataract.

Polarising goggles and sunglasses should always be worn in both natural and artificial sunlight. The damaging effects should be clearly explained to clients.

POLYMORPHIC LIGHT ERUPTION

Certain individuals react adversely to ultraviolet exposure and develop skin eruptions. The reaction occurs a few hours after exposure. There is reddening of the skin and the development of hard, itchy papules and scaling. The reaction will clear in 2–6 days, providing the skin is not exposed to further radiation.

PHOTOSENSITISATION

Certain drugs and cosmetics will produce photosensitisation in individuals who expose themselves to the sun. A painful itchy rash develops which may be followed by pronounced permanent pigmentation. A list of these drugs appears on page 160.

DAMAGE TO THE IMMUNE SYSTEM

Ultraviolet radiation reduces the effectiveness of the immune system. Disturbances and reduction in the number of certain lymphocytes occur as a result of exposure to ultraviolet radiation (including UVA sunbeds). These changes, both cutaneous and systemic, diminish the response of the immune system to infections.

AGGRAVATION OF CERTAIN SKIN CONDITIONS

This occurs as a result of UV exposure, eg eczema and systemic lupus erythematosus is exacerbated.

CONTRA-INDICATIONS TO SUNBED AND SOLARIUM TREATMENTS

1 Individuals who burn easily.
2 Individuals who do not tan easily in the sun, as these individuals have no protection, there is an increased risk of skin damage (types 1 and 2).
3 Those suffering from skin disorders aggravated by sunlight, such as eczema, dermatitis, vitiligo and chloasma.
4 Those who are unwell with colds, fever and high temperature.
5 Those with migraine, headache, faintness.
6 Those with cold sores (herpes simplex).
7 Wounds or recent scars.
8 Heart and blood pressure disorders.
9 Those undergoing or having been treated with deep X-ray therapy.
10 Those with multiple naevi or those with a naevus showing changes in size, pigmentation or inflammation, or anyone with a previous history of skin cancer.
11 Those taking drugs which may produce photosensitisation, these include:

antibiotics	gold injections
tranquillisers	insulin
steroids	thyroid extract
diuretics	quinine
birth control pills	blood pressure tablets

There may be other sensitising drugs; always seek a doctor's advice if clients are taking any medication.

12 Those on long-term immunosuppression drugs.
13 Ultraviolet exposure during pregnancy may result in uneven pigmentation (chloasma).
14 Certain treatments should not be carried out in conjunction with ultraviolet treatment, namely, epilation, waxing and infrared before ultraviolet exposure as it increases sensitivity. (However, infrared given after ultraviolet exposure will reduce the reaction.)

DANGERS OF ULTRAVIOLET EXPOSURE

1 Overdose causing sunburn.
2 Shock from faulty apparatus.
3 Skin ageing and skin cancer.
4 Eye damage – conjunctivitis, keratitis and cataract.
5 Impairment of the immune function.
6 Polymorphic light eruption.
7 Photosensitisation.

FACTORS WHICH DETERMINE THE INTENSITY OF THE REACTION

The erythema reaction of a client will depend on many factors.

THE SENSITIVITY OF THE CLIENT

The reaction of different clients to ultraviolet varies considerably, as shown in the list of skin types (see page 153). The sensitivity of the skin also varies on different parts of the body. Exposed surfaces are less sensitive than those that are normally covered by clothing. The extensor aspects are generally less sensitive than the flexor aspects. A patch test should always be used to determine the client's sensitivity if using mercury vapour lamps. When using sunbeds, the manufacturer's instructions should be carefully followed; first doses should be reduced for sensitive clients.

THE OUTPUT OF THE LAMP OR SUNBED

It is necessary to test the output of every new lamp, and all lamps should be tested at intervals to ensure that there is no change in their output. The object of the test is to find the average dose required to produce an E1 at 36 inches; therefore, the test should be carried out on several individuals. An area of the body which has not been exposed to sunlight is selected and three small areas exposed for $\frac{1}{2}$ minute, 1 minute, $1\frac{1}{2}$ minutes.

When the correct doses on different individuals have been found, the average is taken as the standard dose. Again this is not necessary when using sunbeds. Sunbeds are designed to produce a required reaction at a set distance in a certain time. Tubes should be replaced regularly and if damaged in order to maintain output.

THE DURATION OF EXPOSURE

The duration of exposure will have an effect on the reaction. The longer the time, the greater the reaction at constant distance.

THE DISTANCE BETWEEN THE LAMP OR TUBES AND THE CLIENT

The nearer the lamp, the greater the reaction at constant timing (see law of inverse squares, page 139) which must be considered when changing the distance of the lamps. Again this does not apply to sunbeds where distance is constant.

THE ANGLE AT WHICH THE RAYS STRIKE THE PART (ANGLE OF LAMP)

The angle at which the rays strike the skin affects the dosage. According to the *cosine law*, maximum absorption takes place when the rays strike the skin at right angles. Sunbeds are designed with reflectors to focus the rays on the area and angles cannot be changed.

PREVIOUS EXPOSURE OF THE AREA

An exposure should not be repeated until the previous erythema has faded, as until this occurs sensitivity is increased. When the erythema has faded, there will be a thickening of the skin. It is, therefore, necessary to increase exposure in order to repeat the reaction on the same area of skin. If there has been marked peeling, the exposure should be decreased.

Infrared irradiation applied before exposure to ultraviolet radiation increases the erythema reaction. Infrared applied after ultraviolet reduces the effects. Simultaneous irradiation with both types of ray does not affect the reaction.

PRECAUTIONS

1 On the first consultation, discuss the following with the client:
   (a) Her skin type, ie is she fair, medium or dark skinned.
   (b) Her reaction to sunlight, ie does she go red and never tan, go red first then tan, or does she rarely go red but tan easily.
   (c) Ask when she received her last exposure to sunlight.
      The timing of the first dose will depend on these factors.
2 Check for contra-indications.
3 Explain the procedure to the client; show her the switch, timer, release button and other facilities.
4 Explain the importance of wearing the goggles provided.
5 Explain the importance of not exceeding the treatment time.
6 Always maintain high standards of hygiene.
   (a) The client must shower, both for cleanliness and to remove lotions and perfumes.
   (b) Provide a disposable floor covering for each client.
   (c) Clean the sunbed before and after treatment with detergent recommended by manufacturer.
7 Check the reaction to the previous dose.

TREATMENT TECHNIQUE

MACHINE

1 Ensure that the sunbed is in good working order.
2 Check and set the switch, timer, etc.

3 Clean the bed with a disinfecting detergent recommended by the manufacturer.
4 Place a clean disposable floor covering for each client.
5 Provide clean towels for each client.
6 Provide clean goggles for each client.
7 Ensure that the sunroom is well ventilated.

CLIENT

1 Check for contra-indications.
2 Remove all make up.
3 Remove all jewellery.
4 Shower using non-perfumed soap to remove perfume, cologne, lotions and ointments as these may produce photosensitisation.
5 Ensure that the skin is dry.
6 Remove contact lenses.
7 Wear protective goggles (curved polarising).
8 Cover hair, particularly coloured and bleached hair.
9 Protect protruding haemorrhoids.
10 Do *not* apply any suntan oils or lotions.
11 For sunbeds, the first dose should not exceed 15 minutes – do not give a second dose if there was adverse reaction, such as intense irritation, rash or intense erythema. Do not give further treatment until all erythema has subsided.
12 Stay in easy reach of the client and show her how the sunbed works and how to operate the release button. Explain the dangers of not heeding contra-indications and wearing goggles, etc.
13 After each session, advise the client to get up slowly and apply moisturiser to her face and body.
14 Keep a careful record of: the date of treatment, time of treatment and reaction to treatment.

(Dermatologists recommend that exposure to ultraviolet rays should not exceed 10 hours per year – two courses of 10 half-hour sessions.)

Mercury vapour lamps

These lamps are rarely found in the beauty salon. However, therapists should be aware of the precautions necessary should they be encountered. These lamps may be table or floor models. They have a U-shaped quartz tube containing argon and mercury. This is placed in the centre of a parabolic reflector. The lamp has an on/off switch and a starter button. (This start button activates a step up transformer to increase the voltage and is necessary to ionise the argon.) There is also a variable resistance which is used to increase the current flow as the output of the burner decreases. The radiation from these lamps include UVA, UVB, some UVC, visible and infrared.

They are used for localised treatments of ultraviolet, eg to the face for treatment of acne and to the head for treatment of alopecia. Great care has to be taken when using these lamps. A patch test must be carried out to determine the skin sensitivity. The angle and distance of the lamp must be measured. According to the cosine law, rays should fall at 90 degrees for maximum penetration. The time of the treatment must be recorded. The progression of treatment must be carefully calculated. (These procedures are described clearly on page 166).

PROCEDURE

PREPARATION OF THE CLIENT

1 The sensitivity of client's skin and its reaction to UVL must be calculated using the patch test (see page 165). This should be carried out two or three days before treatment commences. If there is no adverse reaction, the treatment can be carried out.
2 Sit the client in a comfortable position.
3 Clean the face to remove any make up and sebum.
4 Carefully cover all areas not receiving treatment (a note should be made of covering as the same area must be covered each time).
5 Pin her hair back off her face.
6 Apply a thin film of petroleum jelly to eyelids and lips.
7 Cover the eyelids with small pieces of cotton wool to prevent the penetration of rays. This can be stuck on with petroleum jelly. (Goggles are too big and leave unsightly white circles – owl eyes.)
8 Position the lamp centrally with the surface parallel to the part.
9 Measure the chosen distance usually 50 cm (18 in). This must be recorded and measured accurately each time.
10 Remove the cover from the lamp or part and time the irradiation accurately (the timing will depend on the result of the patch test). The rays should strike the part at 90 degrees for maximum penetration.
11 At the end of the treatment, cover the area quickly.
12 If the lamp is no longer required switch it off.
13 Remove cotton wool and petroleum jelly.
14 Explain the effects expected to the client; ask the client to note the time erythema first appeared.

15 The next exposure time will be calculated according to the client's reaction (see page 166); to repeat an E2 add 50 per cent of the previous dose.

LAMP

I Switch the lamp on 5 minutes before treatment commences to allow it to reach maximum intensity.
2 Cover the lamp or the part to prevent radiation (a dark cloth is used over the surface of lamp).

WHEN TREATING THE FACE

The front of the face may be exposed on the first treatment and each side of the face may be exposed on alternate treatments.

WHEN TREATING THE BODY

The front may be exposed on the first treatment and the back exposed on the next treatment.

PATCH TEST

The patch test should be carried on the thigh or any other hidden area of the skin.

Figure 7.16 *Exposure time for the patch test*

Expose I for 30 seconds
Expose I and 2 for 30 seconds
Expose I, 2, 3 for 30 seconds

PROCEDURE

I Clean the skin to ensure that it is free from grease which would act as a barrier.
2 Cut out *three* holes of different size or shape in a piece of lint.
3 Place this on the area where the skin test is to be taken then cover. Cover all surrounding skin with towels.
4 Choose the distance for exposure, eg 46–92 cm.
5 Remove the cover from the smallest hole and expose for 30 seconds.

6 Remove the cover from the second hole and expose both holes for 30 seconds.

7 Remove the cover from the third hole and expose all the holes for a further 30 seconds.

The first hole will now have received $1\frac{1}{2}$ minutes, the second hole 1 minute, and the third hole 30 seconds. The client should carefully observe the reaction and should return the following day for the check up.

For the first degree erythema (E1) slight reddening, which fades in 24 hours is the desired reaction; therefore, the hole that gives this reaction has obtained the correct timing. This treatment should commence using this timing – this timing will give first degree erythema:

$$E2 \text{ is } E1 \times 2\frac{1}{2}$$

To repeat dosage:

To repeat E1 add 25 per cent of the previous dose.
To repeat E2 add 50 per cent of the previous dose.
To repeat E3 add 75 per cent of the previous dose.

Should it be necessary to change the distance of the lamp for any reason, a new dosage must be calculated using the following:

$$\text{New dose} = \frac{\text{old dose} \times \text{new distance}^2}{\text{old distance}^2}$$

To maintain the same dosage at a new distance, using the law of inverse squares.

- If the *distance* is divided by 2 (halved) the *timing* is divided by 4 (quartered).
- If the *distance* is multiplied by 2 the *timing* is multiplied by 4.

Local council regulations in relation to infrared and ultraviolet treatments

Any salon offering infrared or ultraviolet treatments must adhere to the local authority regulations.

CONSTRUCTION OF EQUIPMENT

The collapse of any ultraviolet tanning equipment may give rise to electric shock, fire, or direct physical injury. Equipment should, therefore, be of adequate mechanical strength and rigidity. Lamps should be adequately protected by embedding the lamps within reflectors, or by covering them with a grille mesh.

LAYOUT

- To facilitate rapid entrance or exit from a cubicle containing the equipment, any door should be fitted so that its opening cannot be impeded and must be able to be opened from the outside. Equipment must be designed for easy release by the user.
- Ensure adequate ventilation is provided to prevent a build up of ozone and to ensure that heat generated by the bed is adequately dissipated.
- If the ultraviolet tanning equipment is not in individual cubicles, then suitable screens or curtains should be provided to prevent unnecessary exposure to other persons.

WASHING FACILITIES

Showering/washing facilities should be provided for hygiene reasons.

CLEANING THE EQUIPMENT

Surfaces that come into contact with client should only be cleaned with the appropriate cleaning agents. Other agents may damage or form a film on the acrylic surface: they may be toxic or inflammable or could sensitise the skin of the client.

EXPOSURE

The operator should ensure that as far as it is practical, each client is advised of a suitable exposure regime, taking into account skin types, previous exposures and enhanced sensitivity. A good quality reliable automatic time switch should be carefully pre-set to terminate the exposure.

PROTECTIVE EYE WEAR

The excessive exposure of a person's eyes will result in eye damage. Provide the special goggles, but ensure they are thoroughly cleaned between each client to eliminate the risk of eye infections.

MAINTENANCE

Records should be kept by the operator of all servicing and these should be available on the premises. Servicing and repair must be carried out by a qualified electrician in accordance with manufacturers instructions. Faulty equipment must not be used. All parts must be replaced by the exact same model.

STAFF TRAINING

The operator should ensure that properly trained staff are available to provide adequate advice, supervision and assistance to clients.

SUMMARY

- The electromagnetic spectrum is made up of bands of different wave lengths and frequencies. Infrared radiation and ultraviolet radiation are part of the spectrum; they lie on either side of visible light.
- Infrared rays are used to heat body tissues.
- Ultraviolet rays are used to tan the skin.
- All rays travel in straight lines until they meet a new medium where they may be refracted, reflected or absorbed.
- Refraction means the bending of rays towards or away from the normal as they enter a new medium.
- Reflection means that rays will reflect off certain surfaces; a greater proportion of rays are reflected from white surfaces than from dark-black surfaces.
- Absorption means that rays are absorbed by certain mediums; they do not pass through. When giving infrared or UVL treatments, rays must be absorbed to produce and effect (law of Grotthus). The amount of absorption depends on three factors:
  1 The wave length and frequency of rays.
  2 The type of medium.
  3 The angle at which the rays strike the part.
- The cosine law describes the way that intensity is governed by the angle of incidence. The cosine law states that the intensity at a surface varies with the cosine of the angle of incidence.
- The intensity at surface depends on:
  1 The intensity of the lamp.
  2 The distance between the lamp and the skin.
  3 The angle at which the rays strike the part.

- Rays should strike the part at 90 degrees for maximum intensity, absorption and effect.

- The law of inverse squares governs intensity in relation to distance. The law of inverse squares states that the intensity from a point source varies inversely with the square of the distance from the source. If you halve the distance, you must quarter the time. If you double the distance, you quadruple the time.

- Both infrared lamps (non-luminous) and radiant heat lamps (luminous) emit infrared rays, the difference lies in their wave length. See page 141 for the differences.

DANGERS OF INFRARED TREATMENT

1 burns;
2 shock;
3 headache;
4 faintness;
5 eye damage;
6 chill.

Note: Always carry out a skin sensitivity test before applying infrared to the body. The client must be able to distinguish between hot and cold. Use two test tubes, one with hot water and the other with cold water. Instruct the client to close her eyes. Touch the area to be irradiated with either the hot or cold test tube and ask the client to say if it feels hot or cold. A failure to identify the hot or cold test tube means that treatment should not be carried out.

ULTRAVIOLET

- Ultraviolet rays are used for tanning the body and for certain conditions, such as acne and psoriasis. Ultraviolet rays are divided into three bands according to their wave length:

  UVA – the longest wave length, penetrates down to the dermis.
  UVB – middle wave length, penetrates to stratum basale.
  UBC – shortest wave length, penetrates the stratum corneum.

- Emission of ultraviolet from natural sunlight include all three, but all the UVC and some UVB are filtered out in the atmosphere and do not reach the earth's surface.

- UVC are dangerous and destructive rays. They destroy bacteria and are known as abiotic or germicidal.

- UVB rays are burning rays. They are responsible for sunburn due to overexposure. Long-term or intense exposure to UVB can cause skin cancers.

- At one time it was thought that UVA rays would tan without producing harmful effects. However, they penetrate more deeply into the skin and damage the connective tissue in the dermis, damaging collagen and elastin fibres; this causes ageing and wrinkling of the skin. There is also increasing evidence that intense and over exposure to UVA can cause certain skin cancers.
- Artificial UVL is produced by lamps and tubes found in solariums and sunbeds.
- High pressure mercury vapour lamps emit UVA, UVB and small amounts of UVC as well as visible rays and some infrared.

SOLARIUMS

- These contain elements emitting infrared and tubes emitting UVL. All UVC and most UVB are filtered out of these beds.

SUNBEDS

- These are composed of a collection of long tubes which emit mainly UVA and may also emit very small amounts of UVB.
- Exposure to artificial sunlight will produce some beneficial effects on the body. However, great care must be taken as over or prolonged exposure will have very undesirable effects. (These are fully discussed on page 155.)
- Contra-indications to use of sunbeds must be very carefully studied (see page 160).
- Hygiene precautions when using sunbeds:

  1 Clients should shower and dry before use.
  2 The sunbed should be cleaned with a recommended detergent before and after treatment.
  3 Provide a disposable floor covering.
  4 Provide clean disinfected goggles.
  5 Provide clean towels for each client.
  6 Ensure that the room is well ventilated.

- Before exposure discuss with the client:

  1 Her skin type; fair, medium or dark.
  2 Her reaction to sunlight, ie type 1, 2, 3, 4, 5 or 6.
  3 When she received her previous dose.
  4 Check for other contra-indications; particularly ask about any medication being taken.

- Explain the dangers of over exposure or prolonged exposure.
- Guidelines for users and operators of sunbeds:

1 Use of sunbeds should be limited to 2 courses a year.
2 No more than 10 sessions per course.
3 Each session should be timed to produce a barely perceptible erythema 8–24 hours later. The length of time of exposure should not exceed 30 minutes per session.

(Exposure per year should not exceed 10 hours.)

EFFECTS OF ULTRAVIOLET EXPOSURE

1 Erythema.
2 Tanning.
3 Thickening of epidermis.
4 Skin peeling.
5 Production of vitamin D.
6 Abiotic effect of short rays (not present in normal lamps, solariums and sunbeds).
7 General tonic effect.
8 Skin ageing and wrinkling.
9 Cancer forming.
10 Damage to eyes.
11 Polymorphic light eruptions.
12 Photosensitisation.
13 Damage to immune system.
14 Aggravation of certain skin conditions, eg eczema.

● The patch test (determines the skin reaction to certain exposure times). It is required when using mercury vapour lamps, but not necessary when using solariums and sunbeds because of the very small percentage of UVB in these.

QUESTIONS

1 Explain what is meant by
  (a) wave length of rays
  (b) frequency of rays.
2 Define the term 'incidence ray'.
3 Where does the 'angle of incidence' lie?
4 Explain why a stick looks bent when held in water.
5 Define the law of Grotthus.
6 Name *three* factors which affect the amount absorption by a medium.
7 State the law that governs the way intensity is affected by the angle of incidence.
8 State the law that governs intensity in relation to distance.

9 List the *three* factors which will affect the intensity felt by a client receiving infrared treatment.
10 Give *three* differences between luminous and non-luminous infra infrared lamps.
11 Some lamps are manufactured with two elements, one emitting infrared and the other ultraviolet; explain the danger when using these lamps.
12 Why must a sensitivity test be carried out before an infrared treatment?
13 Explain the procedure for carrying out a sensitivity test.
14 Give the *two* factors that govern the choice of

distance when giving infrared treatments.

15 Explain why it is desirable for rays to strike the part at 90 degrees.

16 Give *three* ways in which vasodilation is produced during heat treatments.

17 Explain why blood pressure will fall when giving heat treatments.

18 Explain why the heart rate increases.

19 Explain why sweating is induced during heat treatments.

20 Explain why the following are contra-indications to infrared treatments:
    (a) heart conditions;
    (b) thrombosis;
    (c) headaches;
    (d) recent exposure to UVL.

21 Give *four* dangers of infrared irradiation.

22 List *six* precautions to be taken when giving infrared treatments.

23 List the three bands of rays in ultraviolet light.

24 Discuss the wave length and compare the depth of penetration of the skin by each band.

25 List six contra-indications to ultraviolet irradiation.

26 Explain the procedure when preparing a sunbed for use.

27 Give three questions that would be asked of a client to determine the length of first exposure.

28 Give three beneficial effects and three detrimental effects of exposure to UVL.

29 Explain how and why tanning of the skin is one effect of exposure to UVL.

30 Give the exposure guidelines to follow for operators and users of sunbeds.

31 In order to produce the same effect on the skin when using an ultraviolet mercury vapour lamp if the distance is halved, how would the timing change?

Heat therapy

Figure 8.1   *A sauna in use*

Objectives

After you have studied this chapter, you will be able to:

1 Differentiate between the methods of giving general heat and local heat to the body.
2 List the effects of heat on the body.
3 Explain the contra-indications to heat on the body.
4 Discuss the advantages and disadvantages of steam baths and steam rooms.
5 Explain the uses of steam baths and steam rooms.
6 Select either a steam bath or steam room and treat the client paying due consideration to maximum efficiency, comfort, safety and hygiene.
7 Briefly explain the production of dry heat in a sauna.
8 Describe the temperature range and seating advice suitable for a client using the sauna for the first time.
9 List the dangers of sauna bath treatment.
10 Treat the client using a sauna bath, paying due consideration to maximum efficiency, comfort, safety and hygiene.
11 Briefly describe the facial steamer.
12 Describe the uses of facial steamers.
13 Explain the danger of facial steamers.
14 Treat the client paying due consideration to maximum efficiency, comfort, safety and hygiene.
15 Indicate the uses of wax treatments to identified areas of the face and body.
16 List the contra-indications to wax treatments in the following areas:
    (a) hands and feet;
    (b) body;
    (c) face.
17 Prepare a wax bath and bring to the correct temperature.
18 Treat the client with wax to hands and feet; to the body; and to the face paying due consideration to maximum efficiency, comfort, safety and hygiene.
19 Describe the care and maintenance of wax baths.

Figure 8.1 is a photograph of a sauna bath; this is one method of applying general heat to the body. Many forms of heat therapy are available to the beauty therapist, and choice is determined by availability, client preference and suitability. All forms of heat produce similar effects; the treatment is particularly beneficial when combined with other treatments as part of a routine. It is mainly used before other treatments as it increases tissue response.

Heat therapy is used for the following reasons:

1 To heat the body prior to other treatments.
2 To induce muscle relaxation.
3 For relief of pain.

Methods of heat application

1 Sauna baths.
2 Steam baths.
3 Infrared lamps and tunnels (discussed fully on page 143).
4 Wax baths.
5 Impulse and ordinary showers.
6 Whirlpool baths.
7 Foam baths.
8 Jacuzzi.

EFFECTS OF HEAT ON THE BODY

(For a detailed explanation see page 143).
1 A general rise in body temperature.
2 An increase in blood flow to the area due to vasodilation giving hyperaemia and erythema.
3 An increase in the heart rate/pulse rate.
4 A lowering of blood pressure.
5 An increase in the metabolic rate; therefore, there is an increased demand for oxygen and nutrients and increased output of waste products.
6 Relaxation of muscles.
7 Mild heat has a soothing effect on sensory nerve endings, but intense heat is irritating to sensory nerve endings.
8 Increased activity of sweat glands (diaphoretic effect).

Heat may be applied generally or locally and the extent of the effects will be dependent on:

1 The duration of heat application.
2 The intensity or degree of the heat.
3 The depth of absorption.
4 The size of area being heated.

METHODS OF APPLYING GENERAL HEAT TO THE BODY

1 Sauna.
2 Steam baths, eg Turkish and Roman baths.
3 Jacuzzi.
4 Infrared tunnels.
5 Wax applied to the body.
6 Various forms of showers.

METHODS OF APPLYING LOCAL HEAT

1 Infrared and radiant heat lamps.

2 Paraffin wax to specific areas.

3 Whirlpool baths.

CONTRA-INDICATIONS TO GENERAL HEAT THERAPY

1 Areas of defective sensation and hypersensitive skins.

2 Heart conditions and blood pressure disorders.

3 Thrombosis or phlebitis.

4 Bronchitis, asthma, hay fever or heavy colds and fevers.

5 Migraine and headache.

6 Skin disorders, such as eczema and psoriasis, may be helped by wet heat (with medical approval).

7 Diabetes.

8 Epilepsy.

9 After a heavy meal.

10 Under the influence of alcohol or drugs.

11 Later stages of pregnancy.

12 First 1–2 days of a period, especially if it is heavy.

13 Severe exhaustion.

14 Recent over exposure to UVL, eg sunburn.

Steam treatments

- Steam may be applied to the body using steam baths or steam rooms. It may be applied to the face by means of facial steamers.

- Steam treatments applied to the body promote relaxation, have a deep cleansing effect and make the tissues more receptive to following treatments.

- Steam is used on the face to soften the skin for deep cleansing and to aid the absorption of creams, oils and masks.

Figure 8.2   *A steam bath in use*

The steam bath

This bath is designed for individual treatments. It is a cabinet made of moulded fibreglass in which the client sits. It contains a trough with a heating element; water poured into the trough is heated making steam. The trough is placed underneath an adjustable seat which allows the client to sit comfortably with her head outside the bath. There are usually three controls: a main switch, a timer and temperature gauge. The water is heated forming steam, this condenses within the bath and the air is saturated with very high humidity of around 95 per cent.

The steam room

This is a room which is supplied with steam from a boiler. Several people may use the steam room together. Some complexes based on Turkish baths have several rooms with increasing temperatures. Clients start with the lowest temperature and progress through to the highest. The steam bath has several advantages over the steam room. However, group treatments in steam rooms are more sociable occasions.

Advantages of the steam bath over the steam room

1 The client does not feel claustrophobic because her head is out of the bath.
2 The clients breathe normal air and not steam.
3 The hair remains neat and tidy and does not get wet.
4 The bath offers privacy for the client.
5 The temperature can be adjusted to suit the individual.
6 The initial cost and the running cost is low compared with a steam room.
7 It takes up little space and can be accommodated in most saloons.

Uses

- To prepare client for further treatment.
- To induce relaxation.
- For deep cleansing.

Effects of steam heat

1 A general rise in body temperature.
2 An increase in circulation due to vasodilation giving hyperaemia and erythema.

3 The heart/pulse rate increases.

4 Superficial capillaries and vessels dilate; therefore, there is a fall in blood pressure.

5 An increase in cell metabolism.

6 Stimulation of sweat glands with increased sweating and elimination of waste. There may be a temporary loss of body fluid due to sweating, but this is soon adjusted by drinking water.

7 The increased circulation and rise in temperature promotes muscle relaxation.

8 The mild heat soothes sensory nerve endings.

9 The superficial layer of the skin is softened and is removed more easily improving tone and texture.

CONTRA-INDICATIONS

1 Heart and circulatory conditions.

2 High or low blood pressure.

3 Thrombosis and phlebitis.

4 Headaches, migraines, dizziness, faintness.

5 Skin diseases.

6 Athlete's foot and verrucas.

7 Diabetics, epileptics.

8 Any chest conditions, eg asthma, bronchitis.

9 First days of menstruation.

10 Pregnancy.

11 After a heavy meal or drinking alcohol.

12 Clients on low calorie slimming diets.

DANGERS

1 Over heating causing fainting or dizziness.

2 Burns from touching the hot metal trough.

3 Cross-infection of micro-organisms.

PRECAUTIONS

1 Ensure good standards of hygiene as moist heat is an ideal breeding ground for micro-organisms. Wipe over the whole bath with sterilising detergent before and after treatment. Cover the seat and floor with towels that are boiled after use or disposed of.

2 Check the power supply and terminals are correctly switched on.

3 Check that the trough is full of distilled water.

4 Protect the client from direct contact with metal and steam using a towel.

5 Remove jewellery, glasses, contact lenses, etc.
6 Check for contra-indications.
7 Ensure that the client takes a shower before and after treatment.
8 Explain the treatment to the client and demonstrate how to open the door and get out of the bath.
9 Wrap a towel around her neck to prevent steam escaping.
10 Stay within calling distance of the client and observe her frequently.

TREATMENT TECHNIQUE

Figure 8.3   *Preparation of a steam bath*

PREPARATION OF THE BATH BEFORE THE CLIENT ARRIVES

1 Wipe over with sterilising detergent.
2 Fill the trough with water.
3 Protect the seat with a towel and ensure that the client is protected from contact with metal or direct steam.
4 Place a towel over the aperture to prevent loss of steam.
5 Turn on the main switch and bath switch.
6 Turn the controls to maximum until the water is heating and then adjust the temperature and timer (50–55°C) the bath will take around 15 minutes to heat from cold.

PROCEDURE

1 Supply the client with a gown and paper slippers.
2 Remove all jewellery, glasses, contact lenses, etc.
3 Check for contra-indications.

4 Explain the treatment to the client and show her how to enter and leave the steam bath/room.
5 Help the client into the shower.
6 After the shower, help the client into the bath; make sure that she is comfortable; close the door.
7 Place a towel around the client's neck over the aperture.
8 Keep in verbal contact throughout, reassure the client and ask her to report any discomfort.
9 Treatment time is 15–20 minutes.
10 Help the client from the bath and into the shower.
11 Advise the client to use a friction rub to aid desquamation and improve skin texture.
12 The client should now rest for 20–30 minutes or receive further treatments *but not exercise.*

Sauna baths

These baths are pine wood log cabins heated by electric stoves. They are manufactured in various sizes, from a single person sauna up to large cabins for 10–14 people. In Scandinavian countries, they are found indoors and outdoors. The larger the sauna, the more expensive it will be to run as it will require more heat output from larger stoves.

The walls of the cabin are constructed of well-insulated panels of pine wood. Pine wood allows the interchange of air and absorbs moisture. This will reduce the humidity inside the cabin giving a dry heat. The heat is provided by electric stoves, which heat non-splintering stones placed on top of the stove. Slatted wooden benches are arranged inside the sauna for sitting or lying down. There is an air inlet near the floor and an outlet near the ceiling. As the air in the sauna is heated, it rises by convection; therefore, the sauna is hotter on the upper benches than on the lower benches. The air moisture is absorbed by the walls, making humidity very low at around 10 per cent. This humidity can easily be increased by pouring water on the stones; this boils making steam. Because the humidity in the sauna is low, sweat from the body evaporates quickly cooling the body, therefore, high temperatures can be tolerated in the sauna. The temperature in the sauna may range from 50°C to around 120°C. A temperature range between 60–80°C is recommended for clients unfamiliar with sauna baths. This can be increased as the client's tolerance increases. The thermometer should always be checked for the temperature and the hygrometer should be checked for humidity before the commencement of treatment. These are found on a wall inside the cabin. The temperature should range from 60–80°C and the humidity should range from 50–70 per cent.

The choice between steam and sauna as a pre-heating treatment depends very much on the client's preference; there are certain differences to consider (see page 183).

USES

- Mainly used as a preheating treatment.
- To induce relaxation.
- For deep cleansing.

EFFECTS

1 A general rise in body temperature.
2 An increase in circulation.
3 The heart rate increases.
4 Superficial capillaries dilate; therefore, there is a fall in blood pressure.
5 Erythema is produced.
6 An increase in cell metabolism.
7 Increased sweating with elimination of waste (diaphoretic effect).
8 Produces relaxation.
9 Sedatory effect on nerve endings.
10 If sweating is excessive, it can produce dehydration.
11 The dry heat is irritating and drying to mucous membranes.

CONTRA-INDICATIONS

1 Heart and circulatory conditions.
2 High and low blood pressure.
3 Thrombosis, phlebitis.
4 Headaches, dizziness, migraines, faintness.
5 Skin diseases.
6 Athletes foot, verrucas.
7 Diabetics, epileptics.
8 Chest conditions, eg asthmatics, bronchitis.
9 First days of menstruation.
10 Pregnancy.
11 After heavy meals or alcohol intake.
12 Clients on low calorie diets.

DANGERS

1 Fainting or dizziness if blood pressure falls too low.

2 Dehydration with prolonged and frequent treatments.

3 Dryness and irritation of mucous membranes, eg the throat and nose.

The therapist should always supervise the sauna.

PRECAUTIONS

1 Check the temperature (60–80°C) and humidity (50–70 per cent) before use.

2 Check that the guard around the heating element is secure and in position.

3 The client must shower to remove all make up, perfumes, etc.

4 Ensure that the client removes her contact lenses, glasses and jewellery.

5 Examine the client for contra-indications, particularly the feet for athlete's foot and verrucas.

6 Use disposable slippers and paper on the floor.

7 Observe the client throughout treatment and check the time.

8 Boil towels or robes after each treatment.

9 Scrub the benches and floor thoroughly with special disinfectant for saunas after use.

TREATMENT TECHNIQUE

1 Prepare the sauna before the client arrives. Protect the floor with paper towelling and bench with towels.

2 Explain the procedure to the client and stress that she must come out if she feels dizzy or faint. Check for contra-indications.

3 The client should shower before treatment and remove jewellery, contact lenses and glasses.

4 The client should wear some form of hair protection.

5 The client enters the sauna with or without a towel wrap and wears disposable slippers.

6 Advise the client to sit or lie on the lower benches until she is accustomed to the heat (hot air rises; lower benches are at lower temperature).

7 Small amounts of water may be sprinkled on the stones from time to time to increase the humidity (this should not be overdone).

8 Treatment time will depend on the tolerance of the client. The first treatment could be up to 5 minutes, increasing to 14 minutes or 20 minutes as the tolerance is built up.

9 Warm or cold showers may be taken during the course of the treatment.

10 The client must always shower after a sauna.

11 Rest after treatment or continue with other treatments, eg massage or vacuum suction, but no exercise.

12 Scrub benches and floor thoroughly with special disinfectants.

Table 1 *Differences between steam baths and saunas*

Steam	Sauna
Moist heat, humidity 95 per cent.	Dry heat, humidity 50–70 per cent.
Atmospheric air is inhaled, therefore more suitable for clients with mild respiratory problems.	Hot, dry air is inhaled which may irritate the mucous membranes.
Easily adjusted to the tolerance of individual clients.	Usually communal, therefore difficult to adjust to the needs of individual clients.
Not claustrophobic as the head is free.	May be claustrophobic.
Not as damaging to hair which is outside.	May damage hair, particularly permed or coloured hair.
Ensures privacy of the client.	Lacks privacy if communal.
Inexpensive to run but may be less profitable as only one client can be treated.	Expensive to run but may be more profitable as many clients may be treated at one time.
Comfortable for most clients.	Less comfortable for the older, less mobile clients or those with sensitive skins.

Facial steamers

Figure 8.4 *A rigid arm vapourizer for facial steam treatment*

Steam may be applied to the face using floor standing or table facial steamers. Some steamers deliver steam only, while others deliver steam and ozone. (Ozone is known to be damaging to the respiratory tract and is not medically recommended. Although only very small amounts are produced by vapour/ozone steamers and the timing of the treatment is reduced to 5 minutes, therapists should take care when giving this treatment.) The facial steamer consists of a tank with a heating element. This is filled with distilled water, which is heated producing steam. This steam passes into a tube, which is directed at the client's face. If it produces ozone, the steamer will contain a high pressure mercury vapour tube producing ultraviolet rays. This converts the oxygen in the air into ozone ie O_2 is converted into O_3. Facial steamers produce heating with high humidity.

USES

1 To soften superficial keratinised cells and build up of sebum, prior to desquamation and deep cleansing.
2 To aid absorption and enhance the effect of creams, oils and masks, etc; used to improve the condition of dry and normal or mature skins.
3 To promote relaxation.
4 To prepare the skin for further treatments.
5 To aid healing of blemished or pustular seborrhoeic skins.

EFFECTS

1 The heat raises the temperature of the area.
2 The circulation is increased due to vasodilation, giving hyperaemia and erythema.
3 The heat induces muscle relaxation.
4 Mild heat is soothing to sensory nerve endings.
5 The heat increases the metabolic rate.
6 Sweat glands are stimulated producing more sweat (diaphoretic effect).
7 Sebaceous glands are stimulated, opening pores and aiding the release of blockages.
8 If ozone is used, it has a bactericidal effect.

CONTRA-INDICATIONS

1 Highly vascular florid or couperosed skin.
2 Highly sensitive skin (low heat tolerance) or telangiectasis.
3 Very dry or weathered skin.
4 Rosacea.
5 Abrasions or chapped skins.

Dangers

1 Burns if the steamer falls over on to the client.
2 Shock if the apparatus is faulty.
3 Damage to the respiratory tract if too much ozone is inhaled.

Precautions

1 Check that there is distilled water in the tank.
2 Switch on for 5–10 minutes before treatment until the vapour is produced.
3 Switch on the ozone after the production of vapour.
4 Cover the client's eyes with damp cotton wool pads.
5 Make sure that the steamer is positioned safely so that it cannot be overturned causing burns.
6 Make sure that the steamer is working correctly and not spitting-out hot water.

Treatment technique

Figure 8.5   *A facial steam treatment*

PREPARATION OF THE CLIENT

1 Place the client in a comfortable, well-supported position.
2 Remove all jewellery and metal.
3 Check for contra-indications.
4 Cover all areas except the face with towels.
5 Cleanse the skin.
6 Explain the procedure to the client.
7 Apply cotton wool pads to the client's eyes.

PROCEDURE

1 Place the machine in stable position and check the plugs and leads.
2 Fill the tank with distilled water.
3 Switch on and allow the steam to build up, then switch on the ozone if required.
4 Position 12–15 inches from the client's face depending on her skin type and tolerance.
5 Time 5–20 minutes depending on the required effect. (If vapour ozone is used, timing should be reduced to 5 minutes and the distance increased to 18 inches.)
6 Switch off and remove the machine to a safe place.
7 Dry the skin and remove the eye pads.
8 Extract any comedones, milia, etc.
9 Follow with other treatments.

Paraffin wax to the hands and feet

Figure 8.6   *A paraffin wax heater – (5 litre capacity)*

Paraffin wax treatment can be used for the face, the whole body or for the hands and feet. When cold, the wax is whitish and solid, but when heated it liquefies and clarifies.

EQUIPMENT

Wax is heated in containers, which vary in size and shape. The larger models have a water jacket and automatic temperature controls. Wax is heated and maintained at a temperature of 45–49°C. The warm wax is applied in layers using a brush or ladle; when treating hands and feet these can be quickly dipped into the wax. Each layer of wax is allowed to dry and become white before the next coat is applied. A build up of six coats is desirable. The area is then wrapped in polythene, grease proof paper or tinfoil and covered with a towel to retain the heat. The application of wax can be messy and care must be taken to cover the floor and clothing before the treatment starts.

USES

1 To relieve pain.
2 To promote relaxation.
3 To soften the skin and cuticles.
4 To increase the circulation.
5 To improve the condition of stiff, arthritic joints. Exercises given after wax may result in increased mobility.

EFFECTS

1 The heat raises the temperature of the area.
2 There is an increase in circulation due to vasodilation, giving hyperaemia and erythema.
3 The heat induces muscle relaxation.
4 The heat soothes sensory nerve endings.
5 The stimulation of sweat glands and more sweat is produced.
6 The stimulation of sebaceous glands thus softening the skin.
7 The moisture/grease in the wax softens the skin and cuticles.
8 An increase in the metabolic rate.

CONTRA-INDICATIONS

1 Skin diseases and disorders, particularly verrucae, athlete's foot and eczema.
2 Cuts and abrasions; small cuts can be covered with a waterproof plaster.
3 Severe bruising or swelling.
4 Any infected areas of cuticle, nails or skin.
5 Undiagnosed painful areas, seek medical advice.
6 Very hairy areas.

DANGERS

Burns of the skin if the temperature is too high, 49°C is the correct temperature. (Use a sugar thermometer if the wax bath is not automatically controlled.)

PRECAUTIONS

1 Cover all areas not receiving treatment.
2 Test the wax on yourself before treatment.
3 Do not hold the part in the wax bath.

TREATMENT TECHNIQUE

PREPARATION OF THE CLIENT

1 Place the client in a well-supported, comfortable sitting position.
2 Check that all jewellery has been removed.
3 Check for contra-indications.
4 Cover the floor and protect the client's clothing.
5 Wash the area thoroughly with warm, soapy water, rinse and dry.
6 Explain the procedure to the client.

PROCEDURE

1 Check the temperature of the wax on yourself and on the client.
2 Hold the part above the bath and apply a thin coat of wax with a brush or ladle and allow the wax to dry. Repeat five or six times until the part is well covered. Work quickly.
3 Cover with polythene, grease proof paper or tinfoil and then wrap in a towel.
4 Leave the wax on for around 20 minutes.
5 Remove the towel and paper and slide off the wax.
6 Pat the area with a tissue to dry.
7 Dispose of wax into a boiler or into a bin.
8 Follow with other treatments.

Paraffin wax to the body

Wax can be applied to the body for the same uses and effects. It is messy and difficult to apply and generally requires an area or room devoted entirely to wax treatments. The therapist must work quickly and deftly to apply a good, even coating, as the wax can cool quickly when applied to large areas.

TREATMENT TECHNIQUE

- Prepare the bed.
- Cover with large bath towels or a blanket.
- Cover this with a large polythene sheet.

PREPARATION OF THE CLIENT

1 The client must shower and dry thoroughly.

2 Check that all jewellery has been removed.
3 Check for contra-indications.
4 Position the client on one side on the bed.
5 Protect the pubic region and gluteal fold with large tissue.
6 Explain the procedure to the client.

PROCEDURE

1 Using a large wax bath containing hot wax at 49°C, paint the client's back with wax. Use a wide brush and work quickly; cover the back and legs with several layers.
2 Turn the client on to her back and paint her front with wax in the same way.
3 Wrap the client in the polythene sheet and then the towel.
4 Leave the client to rest for 20 minutes. (A heat lamp can be used to maintain the heating effect if required.)
5 Unwrap the client and remove the wax from the front; turn the client and remove wax from her back.
6 Follow with a warm shower and other treatments, such as massage.

Paraffin wax to the face

Paraffin wax may be applied to the face as part of a facial routine. Great care must be taken in its application avoiding the eyes, nostrils and mouth.

USES

1 To improve the condition of the dry, dehydrated coarse skin.
2 To stimulate the secretions of sebaceous glands.
3 To improve the condition of mature, ageing skin.
4 To stimulate and cleanse a sluggish skin and remove build up of sebum and dry keratinised cells.
5 To aid the relaxation of facial muscles.

EFFECTS

1 The heat raises the temperature of the area.
2 The circulation is increased due to vasodilation, giving hyperaemia and erythema.
3 The stimulation of sebaceous glands; this releases blockages on a sluggish skin and helps to lubricate the dry, mature skin.
4 An increase in activity of sweat glands.
5 The moisture/grease in the wax will soften the skin.

6 There is an increase in the metabolic rate, which will improve the condition of the skin.

7 The heat soothes sensory nerve endings.

8 The heat induces muscle relaxation.

Contra-indications

1 Any skin disorders or diseases.

2 Skin infections, eg pustular acne.

3 Highly vascular, florid, couperose skins or with telangiectasis.

4 Weathered skin with windburn or sunburn.

5 Low tolerance to heat.

6 Claustrophobic or highly tense, nervous clients.

7 Cuts and abrasions of the skin, eg chapped skin.

Dangers

1 Burning if the temperature of the wax is too high; maintain the heat at 45–49°C. Always test on yourself and on the client before treatment.

2 Spillages of very hot wax; do not move heated baths.

3 Igniting the wax if near a naked flame or hot plate.

Precautions

1 Test the temperature of the wax with a sugar thermometer and test on yourself or the client.

2 Place the wax containers on a stable base away from any flame or hot plates.

3 Check for contra-indications.

4 Explain the treatment to the client.

Treatment technique

PREPARATION OF THE CLIENT

1 Place the client in a well-supported, comfortable position.

2 Check that all jewellery has been removed.

3 Check for contra-indications.

4 Explain the treatment to the client.

5 Cleanse the skin.

6 Cover the hair with a towel or band to the hair line.

7 Protect clothing with towels.

8 Place eye pads over the eyes.

PROCEDURE

1 Place the wax bath on a suitable stable base near the plinth.
2 Protect the working area; cover the floor, plinth and trolley.
3 Check the temperature of the wax on a thermometer (45–49°C), then test it on yourself (the inner wrist is a good area), then test it on the client's neck.
4 Apply the wax quickly to the face and neck using a small brush ($\frac{1}{2}$ or 1 in); continue until a good, even coating has been applied all over (approximately six layers deep; avoid the eyes, nostrils and mouth).
5 Cover the waxed area with polythene or greaseproof paper and then a towel; again avoid the eyes, nostrils and mouth.
6 Leave the client to rest for approximately 20 minutes depending on the skin condition and desired result.
7 Maintain verbal contact throughout; the client should avoid facial movement and so instruct her to lift her hand if she is uncomfortable or in need of assistance or give her a bell to ring.
8 Remove the wax mask; it should lift off easily if the layers are thick enough.
9 Wipe the skin with tissue.
10 Extract comedones if necessary.
11 Cleanse the skin and follow with a facial routine.

CARE AND MAINTENANCE OF WAX

- Wax is supplied as large blocks; these should be covered and kept in a dry cupboard.

- Check the blocks before placing them in the bath, remove any dirt, hairs etc. After use the wax may be disposed of by wrapping in paper and placing in a bin. However, this proves expensive and the wax may be re-used provided it is cleaned and sterilised.

- To clean the wax take a large metal bowl and pour in 2–3 pints of water. Put all the used wax into the bowl. At the end of the day place the bowl on a heating plate and bring to the boil. Boil for over 20 minutes then turn off the heat. Leave the wax overnight; the wax will rise to the top and solidify, the water and other matter will remain underneath. Prise out the wax and scrape all debris from the underside. It may be necessary to remove one-quarter to one-half of the wax. When the wax is clean, it can be re-used in the wax bath.

- Throw away the water and debris in the bowl and wash the bowl thoroughly with hot, soapy water.

● This has been an accepted method of cleaning wax in the past, however, there is some doubt that it meets today's more stringent hygiene conditions. It is more hygenic to dispose of the wax after use.

SUMMARY

STEAM TREATMENT

Steam may be applied using steam baths or steam rooms or using facial steamers. Water is heated forming steam-humidity at 95 per cent.

STEAM BATHS

Steam bath: wet heat
Temperature: 50–55°C
Treatment time: 15–20 minutes

Dangers
1 Over-heating causing fainting and dizziness.
2 Burns from touching the metal trough.
3 Cross-infection of micro-organisms, as these baths are ideal breeding ground.

SAUNA

Sauna: dry heat.
Temperature: 60–80°C building up to 110°C as the tolerance increases
Humidity range: increased by applying water to coals
Cooler on lower shelf, hotter on upper shelf
Treatment time: 5–20 minutes

Dangers
1 Fainting or dizziness.
2 Dehydration.
3 Dryness and irritation of mucous membranes.

FACIAL STEAMERS

Facial steamers: heating with high humidity; water in container is heated and steam delivered to face; some include ozone in treatment
Distance from face: 12–15 in
Treatment time: 5–20 minutes
Treatment time with ozone: 5 minutes only at distance of 18 in

PARAFFIN WAX

Paraffin wax: may be used on the face, body, hands or feet
Temperature of wax: 45–49°C
Treatment time: 20–30 minutes

QUESTIONS

1 List three methods of applying general heat to the body and three methods of applying local heat.
2 Explain why hyperaemia and erythema occur as a result of heat on the tissues.
3 State what happens to the following when the body is heated:
(a) The heart and pulse rate.
(b) The blood pressure.
4 Explain why there is an increase in the activity of sweat glands during heat treatments.
5 List the four factors which influence the extent of the effects when giving heat treatments.
6 Give six advantages of using a steam bath rather than steam room.
7 Give the temperatures recommended for the following treatments:
(a) steam bath;
(b) sauna;
(c) wax application.

8 Explain briefly why the following conditions are contra-indications to heat treatment:
(a) heart and circulatory conditions;
(b) thrombosis;
(c) faintness;
(d) diabetes.
9 Give three dangers associated with sauna treatments.
10 Explain the procedure for preparing the sauna and the client before sauna treatment.
11 The facial steamer may be used for steam only or may include ozone. Give the timing and distance for treatment when using:
(a) steam only;
(b) steam with ozone.
12 List five contra-indications to facial steam treatment.
13 Explain the precautions to be taken before the application of wax treatments.
14 Describe the care and maintenance of paraffin wax.

CHAPTER 9 *Hygiene*

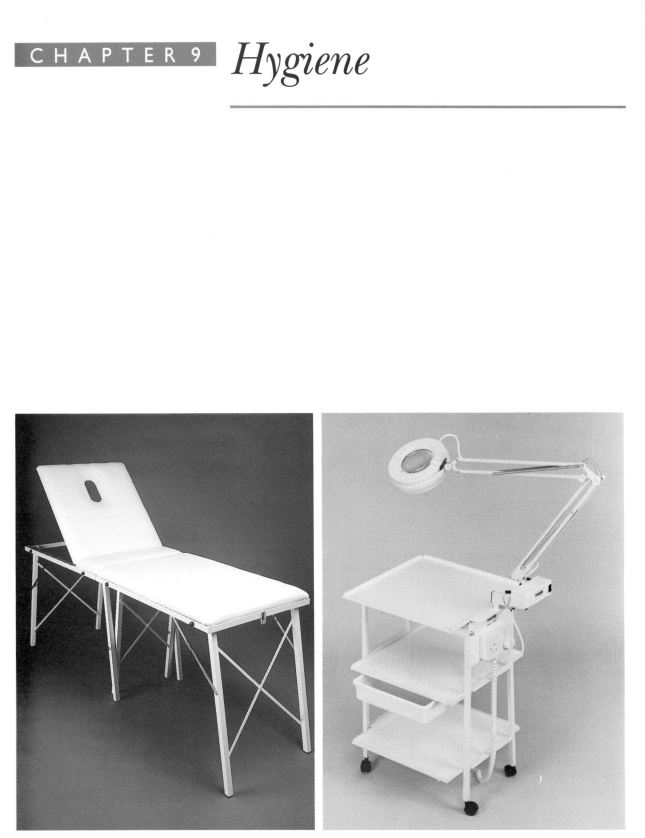

Figure 9.1   *A bed with hard, easy-clean cover; a hygienic trolley*

OBJECTIVES

After you have studied this chapter you will be able to:

1 Distinguish between infection and infestation.
2 Differentiate between bacteria, viruses, fungi and protozoa.
3 List some common diseases caused by each micro-organism.
4 Distinguish between natural immunity and artificial immunity.
5 List the ways in which micro-organisms enter the body.
6 Explain how micro-organisms may be transmitted.
7 List the required conditions for the growth of bacteria.
8 Describe the cause, symptoms and transmission of hepatitis.
9 Describe the cause, symptoms and transmission of HIV which causes AIDS.
10 Distinguish between ectoparasites and endoparasites.
11 Explain the meaning and terminology used in control of micro-organisms.
12 List three methods of sterilisation.
13 Select methods of sterilisation for use in the salon.
14 List a selection of disinfectants available.
15 Select appropriate disinfectants for specific apparatus.
16 Discuss the factors to be considered in maintaining high standards of salon hygiene.
17 Discuss the factors to be considered in maintaining high standards of personal hygiene.
18 Describe the factors to be considered when setting up a salon.

Hygiene deals with the precautions and procedures necessary for maintaining health and preventing the spread of disease. In the beauty salon, the highest priority must be given to preventing infection, cross-infection and infestation. The beauty therapist carries a heavy responsibility for protecting herself, other staff and the clients from the risk of contamination by micro-organisms which cause disease.

Infection

An infection or infectious disease is caused by micro-organisms invading the body. The symptoms and severity of the illness will depend on the type of invading micro-organism and the part of the body affected.

Infestation

An infestation is the invasion of the body by animal parasites, such as lice, worms and flukes; they may live in or on the body. Some parasites merely cause itchy irritation, while others cause serious illness.

Micro-organisms or microbes

There are many different types of micro-organisms present in the environment. The main groups include:

- bacteria;
- viruses;
- fungi, yeasts;
- protozoa.

Micro-organisms entering the body do not always produce disease as the body is continually fighting these pathogens. This ability to fight off disease is known as *resistance*. However, if the invading organisms are in large enough numbers to overcome the body defences, disease and illness will result. There are various kinds of *non-specific resistance*, which are directed against all pathogens.

WAYS IN WHICH THE BODY RESISTS INFECTION (NON-SPECIFIC RESISTANCE)

1 Unbroken skin forms a physical barrier.
2 Mucous membranes, mucus, hairs and cilia help to trap and filter microbes.
3 Saliva washes microbes from teeth and mouths.
4 Tears wash microbes from the eyes.
5 Urine washes microbes from the urethra.
6 Faeces remove microbes from the bowel.
7 The acidic pH of the skin limits growth of bacteria.
8 Sebum produces an oily film which protects the skin.
9 Gastric juices destroy bacteria in the stomach.
10 Various antimicrobial substances are produced by the body in response to infection, eg interferon.
11 Macrophages and granulocytes ingest and destroy micro-organisms by a process of phagocytosis.

The body also produces specific antibodies to destroy a particular antigen. This *specific resistance* to disease is known as *immunity*. Disease will occur if the body has little immunity to the invading microbes, or if the immune system has itself been damaged, as happens with the Human Immunodeficiency Virus (HIV). Immunity is gained as a result of the body coming into contact with an antigen and producing T cells or antibodies to control it. Immunity may be acquired naturally or artificially.

IMMUNITY

NATURAL ACTIVE IMMUNITY

This is obtained when a person comes into contact with a particular microbe and produces antibodies or T cells to repel and control it. These antibodies remain in the body to control future infection. Many infectious diseases occur only once in a lifetime as immunity is lifelong while others may recur as immunity may last for only a few years.

NATURAL PASSIVE IMMUNITY

This involves the transfer of antibodies from an immunised donor to a recipient. Immunity may be passed from mother to baby via the placenta or mother's milk.

ARTIFICIAL ACTIVE IMMUNITY

Artificial immunity can be provided by the use of vaccines. These are prepared from altered or diluted forms of the organism. Once they are introduced into the body, they stimulate the immune system in the same way as an infection, but are not strong enough to cause the disease.

ARTIFICIAL PASSIVE IMMUNITY

Another type of immunisation relies on transferring antibodies from someone who has recovered from that particular disease. The transfer is made via a serum containing the antibodies.

INVASION

Micro-organisms enter the body via many routes:

1 Through broken or damaged skin.
2 Through orifices, such as the nose, mouth, anus, vagina and urethra.
3 Through the eyes and ears.
4 Into hair follicles.
5 Into the blood stream by bloodsucking insects such as mosquitoes and lice.

Some micro-organisms produce immediate symptoms, while others can lie dormant for a long time and attack when the body's immune system is low.

TRANSMISSION

Micro-organisms are transmitted in many ways.

1 By droplet infection; an infected person coughing and sneezing or spitting will expel organisms into the air where they may be inhaled by others.

2 By handling contaminated articles, such as clothing, towels and equipment, when micro-organisms may be transmitted to the handler.

3 Dirty surfaces or dusty atmospheres will contain micro-organisms, which may be inhaled or may enter via the eyes or ears.

4 Organisms present in faeces and urine may be transferred to others if the hands are not thoroughly washed after visiting the toilet.

5 Food may become contaminated by handling with unwashed hands and flies carrying contamination from excreta and rubbish. Water may become contaminated and then organisms will be transmitted through eating and drinking these foods.

6 Organisms may be spread through contact with animals.

7 Through direct contact with others, eg kissing, hand contact or touching.

8 Organisms may be spread through an intermediary host, such as fleas and bloodsucking insects.

9 Sexual intercourse can spread certain organisms which produce venereal diseases.

10 Contaminated blood, if transmitted to another person, can cause serious and, sometimes, fatal illness. Organisms can be transmitted through blood transfusion, infected needles or at any time when the blood of the carrier (infected person) enters the body of the recipient. Hepatitis B and HIV are transmitted in this way, and great care must be taken in the salon to avoid any contact with blood. Needles and ear piercing equipment must be carefully disposed of into 'sharps' boxes. Any blood spots should be dealt with by wearing gloves and using strong disinfectant, eg household bleach.

11 Infection can be caused by the spread of certain organisms within one's own body. These organisms may be harmless in one part of the body, but will produce inflammation in another, eg certain organisms in the intestine are harmless, but if they invade the bladder they produce cystitis.

Bacteria

Bacteria are single cell organisms varying in size from 0.2 to 2.0 μm in diameter. They are found everywhere in the

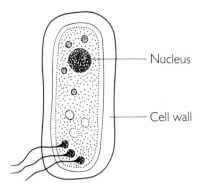

Figure 9.2   *A bacterium*

environment and can be seen through an optical microscope. Many bacteria are harmless and useful to man and are called *non-pathogenic bacteria*. Some are used in the production of food, such as cheese and yoghurt. Others help to dispose of unwanted organic material, such as the breakdown of sewage, rendering it harmless. Some bacteria in the human intestine help to synthesise vitamins K and B_2.

The harmful bacteria which cause disease are known as *pathogenic bacteria* or *pathogens*. Bacteria are the simplest of living organisms, composed of a single cell with cytoplasm surrounded by a protective cell membrane but devoid of organelles. They multiply rapidly by dividing into two, known as *binary fission*. This can occur every 20 minutes and a single bacterium may give rise to 16 million bacteria per day. Some bacteria have whip-like projections on the surface of the cell called flagella which enable the bacteria to move around. Bacteria may be aerobic, requiring oxygen to sustain life, or they may be anaerobic, able to survive without oxygen.

The aerobic variety is found invading surface tissues of the skin and mucous membranes of the respiratory tract. The anaerobic variety is found in the bowel or deep wounds. Some bacteria develop into spores; these can lie dormant for long periods of time and become active when conditions are suitable. Spores develop a hard, thick outer shell which protects the contents and makes them very difficult to destroy. They are more resistant to heat and disinfectants. Higher temperatures and strong chemical disinfectants are required to kill spores.

TYPES OF BACTERIA

Figure 9.3   *Types of bacteria*

Cocci (spherical)   Bacilli (rod-shaped)   Spirochete (spirals)

Bacteria are classified according to their shape:

- Cocci are spherical.
- Bacilli are rod-shaped.
- Spirochetes are spirals or curves.

I *Cocci*. These spherical-shaped bacteria may form clusters known as staphylococci, or they may form chains known as streptococci or they may form pairs known as diplococci. They can cause a wide variety of conditions, such as boils, carbuncles, impetigo, sore throat, meningitis and pneumonia.

2 *Bacilli*. These rod-shaped bacteria cause serious illness, such as diptheria, tuberculosis and typhoid fever.

3 *Spirochetes*. These spiral- or curved-shaped bacteria include spirillium and vibros and cause venereal disease, such as syphilis, and serious disease, such as cholera.

Bacteria cause disease by producing toxins or poisons which are harmful to body cells. The body protects itself against bacterial infection by several methods:

1 By producing antitoxins which neutralise toxins produced by the bacteria.

2 By producing large numbers of white cells, macrophages and granulocytes, which circulate in the blood and which engulf and destroy bacteria.

3 By producing antibodies which attack and destroy the bacteria.

The discovery of penicillin and the development of other antibiotics and antibacterials means that bacterial infections can be brought under control. Antibiotics must be used in adequate doses for at least 5 days. Some antibiotics kill the bacteria directly, while others prevent multiplication of the bacteria.

Bacteria grow and multiply if the conditions are right. These are

1 A food supply.

2 A water supply or moisture.

3 Warmth; pathogenic bacteria favour a body temperature of 37°C. Low temperatures found in the refrigerator or freezer will limit the growth of bacteria, but will not destroy them.

4 Dark conditions; strong ultraviolet light will kill bacteria.

5 Oxygen is required by some bacteria for aerobic respiration, but others are anaerobic and survive without oxygen.

6 Slightly alkaline conditions. (The acidity of the skin (acid mantle), helps to protect against the growth of bacteria.)

Viruses

Viruses are the smallest known infective particles, smaller than bacteria, they can only be seen through an electron microscope. They are between 0.1 and 0.2 μm in size and they vary in shape from spheres, cubes or rods.

They consist of a core of nucleic acid, RNA or DNA, enclosed in a protein shell or capsid. Viruses cannot metabolise or reproduce; they are parasitic, living inside a host cell. Once inside a virus causes the host cell to replicate – make copies of the virus. After

Protein coat

Viral RNA

Figure 9.4   *A virus*

the virus enters the host cell there is a period of 'incubation' – the host cells show no sign of disease. Eventually, the host cell is destroyed and hundreds of new viruses are released which attack other cells. Many cycles of viral spread occur and more and more host cells are affected; eventually typical signs and symptoms of the disease occur. By the time the symptoms appear, the viruses are so numerous that antiviral drugs have limited effect. The body protects itself against viral infection by producing specific antibodies. These will also provide future immunity to some diseases; immunity can be produced artificially to combat some viral infections. Body cells also produce 'interferons' which interfere with the multiplication of viruses.

Antiviral drugs are now available; some prevent the multiplication of viruses while others alter the DNA within the cell, preventing the virus from using it. In this way, the spread of infection is halted. Viral diseases include the common cold, influenza, poliomyelitis, mumps, herpes simplex and zoster, chickenpox, warts, hepatitis and HIV.

Hepatitis and HIV

The two most serious viral infections that could be transmitted between clients or staff and clients in the salon are hepatitis B and HIV, both of which are carried in the blood. Minute amounts of blood or organic material can carry infection, it may not be visible to the naked eye. The correct hygiene procedures must be followed to prevent any possibility of infection (see page 216).

HEPATITIS – INFLAMMATION OF THE LIVER

Hepatitis is caused by viruses or by amoebae. There are three forms of the disease, each having similar symptoms but contracted by different viruses, namely: hepatitis A virus, hepatitis B virus and hepatitis non A and B.

SYMPTOMS OF HEPATITIS

1 Fever.
2 Loss of appetite.
3 Nausea and vomiting.
4 Jaundice (yellow colouring of the skin and whites of the eyes).
5 Pain in the abdomen with tenderness over the liver.
6 Dark urine.

Patients feel very ill for several months and need a long period of convalescence. Patients recover eventually but death may result; death rarely occurs with hepatitis A but is more common with hepatitis B.

HEPATITIS A VIRUS

Hepatitis A virus has a short incubation period of around three weeks. It is contracted through faecal contact due to poor sanitation and poor personal hygiene. It may be contracted by UK residents travelling abroad where faecal-oral contamination is likely and waste disposal may be basic with open sewers, etc. The virus may have already been passed on before the sufferer realises that she is infected as it is most contagious during the incubation period. It does not cause any lasting damage to the liver.

HEPATITIS B VIRUS

This has a long incubation period of around three months. It is transmitted through breaks in the skin or by punctures with contaminated equipment. It may also be transmitted sexually or following transfusion with contaminated blood. Highly infectious mothers usually pass it on to their babies. The virus is detected in blood, saliva, semen and body fluids. High-risk groups are: drug abusers, homosexuals and renal dialysis patients.

The disease is most contagious during the incubation period when a carrier may not be showing any symptoms. There are thousands of symptomless carriers world wide. Hepatitis B can cause lasting chronic liver damage that may result in death.

The particular danger to the beauty therapist and her clients is the transmission of this disease during electrolysis, or on any occasion where blood contamination is likely. Blood, tissue fluid and skin debris may be carried on the needle and transmitted from one client to another or to the therapist by accidental needle stabs.

Disposable 'sterex' needles must always be used in the salon to prevent the spread of this disease. Used needles should be very carefully handled and disposed of in a 'sharp's box', which must be incinerated. Hepatitis B is a particularly resistant virus. Sterilisation using the autoclave and the use of disinfectants, such as 70 per cent isopropyl alcohol and chlorine, are the most effective methods of control.

HEPATITIS NON-A AND NON-B

These have an incubation period of around one month and are distinct from the previous two but produce very similar symptoms. They may be contracted from contaminated food and water or blood transfusions. They can cause inflammation of the liver followed by cirrhosis (scarring of the liver).

Human Immunodeficiency Virus (HIV) which causes aids – acquired immune deficiency syndrome

Aids was first reported in the New England Medical Journal in 1981 and by the end of that year the first case was reported in the United Kingdom. It is a disease which affects both homosexuals and heterosexuals and both males and females.

In 1983 scientists in the United States of America and France isolated the HIV virus which causes AIDS. This virus attacks a group of cells called T4 or the T helper cells which play a part in co-ordinating the action of the immune system.

Following infection with HIV, there may be no immediate symptoms and the incubation period may be up to eight years. There are many thousands of symptomless carriers world wide. The first symptoms are usually fatigue, fever, swollen glands and headaches. After a few weeks these symptoms may disappear.

Some time later the next stage of the disease appears when the glands of the neck, armpit and groin become chronically swollen. During this time the helper T cells which play a key role in antibody production, diminish in number until eventually the body's immune system is destroyed. The body is then defenceless against a wide variety of diseases which include pneumonia, tuberculosis, thrush and Karposi's sarcoma (a deadly skin cancer which produces purple-brownish marks on the skin). The heart, liver and brain may also become affected leading to dementia and death.

This virus has been located in blood, semen, vaginal fluid, tears, saliva and cerebro-spinal fluid, however, to be transmitted the virus must be present in large numbers, these are found only in blood, semen and vaginal secretions.

Ways in which HIV is transmitted:

1 Sexual intercourse with an infected person male to male, male to female or female to male.
2 Through blood exchange from open bleeding cuts and wounds; from contaminated needles or other contaminated instruments piercing the skin.
3 Infected mothers pass it to their babies through the placenta, during birth or through breast feeding.

No cure has been found to date and preventative measures must be taken to avoid spread of the disease. The virus is quite fragile outside the body and can be destroyed by: Autoclaving all contaminated instruments; washing towels, dishes etc at 56°C for ten minutes; cleaning surfaces with 70 per cent alcohol or chlorine bleach; and by soaking blood spills with chlorine bleach for ten minutes.

Fungi

Figure 9.5 *Fungi*

Fungi are larger than bacteria; they may be unicellular, as in yeasts, or multicellular, as in moulds. The cells contain nuclei and other cell components, but do not contain chlorophyll. They obtain their food by secreting enzymes through the cell walls. This digests any organic matter which is then absorbed as liquid food. Fungi may be saprophytes which obtain food from dead organic matter, or parasites, living off plants, animals or humans and feeding off skin and mucous membranes and producing diseases. They reproduce by forming spores. The unicellular fungi and spores are not visible to the naked eye, but the filamentous fungi forming mycelia are visible, eg moulds and mildews.

Fungi require similar conditions to bacteria for growth, ie:

1 A food supply.
2 Damp, moist conditions.
3 Warmth.
4 Oxygen, although some survive for a short time without.

Diseases caused by fungi are:

1 Ringworm:
   (a) Of the foot, tinea pedis (athlete's foot).
   (b) Of the body, tinea corporis.
   (c) Of the head, tinea capitis.
   (d) Of the nail, tinea unguium.
2 Thrush, which is caused by the fungus *Candida albicans.*
3 More serious internal fungal infections of the lungs and heart can be fatal.

Once fungal infections invade the body and grow, antifungal drugs are required to control the infection as the condition will rarely improve without drugs. Some antifungal drugs are applied to the areas, while others are taken by mouth. They destroy the fungal cell wall and the cell dies.

Protozoa

These are the simplest of single-celled animals, slightly bigger than bacteria. Each protozoa is composed of cytoplasm containing a nucleus and organelles surrounded by a cell wall or membrane. They move around by pushing out pseudopodia. Many types are known to exist as parasites on humans, particularly in the bowel. Some are harmless causing few symptoms, while others cause different types of illness, some very serious depending on the organism involved.

Protozoa may be transmitted from contaminated food and water, through sexual contact and by bites from insects. They may infect the bowel causing diarrhoea with general ill health and malaise, or they may cause serious illness, such as sleeping sickness, malaria and amoebic dysentery.

As protozoa are difficult to eradicate, treatment requires antiprotozoal drugs to be given over a long period of time.

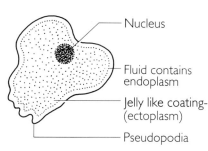

Nucleus

Fluid contains endoplasm

Jelly like coating (ectoplasm)

Pseudopodia

Figure 9.6   *Protozoa*

Animal parasites

Parasites are living organisms that live in or on another living organism and derive their food supply from that host.

● *Ectoparasites* live outside the host, eg lice and fleas.
● *Endoparasites* live inside the host, eg tapeworms or threadworms, roundworms and flukes.

The presence of any parasite on the body is known as an *infestation.*

ECTOPARASITES

Figure 9.7   *Head louse*

Figure 9.8   *Body louse*

Figure 9.9   *Itch mite*

Figure 9.10   *A flea*

HEAD LICE (*Pediculus capitis*)

The head louse is an insect found on the human scalp. It obtains its nourishment by piercing the skin and sucking blood. The adult female is slightly larger than the male, about 2–3 mm long and 1 mm wide. The female lays white, shiny oval shaped eggs called nits; they are cemented to the hair close to the scalp. They take approximately 1 week to mature and can reproduce in another week. The life cycle of a louse lasts for 4–5 weeks, during which time the female will lay around 300 eggs. They cause intense itching and secondary infections may result due to scratching. Lice and nits may be killed by special shampoos or lotions containing insecticide and combing out with a fine tooth comb.

BODY LICE (*Pediculus corporis*)

These are similar but larger than head lice. They obtain nutrients by sucking blood and laying eggs in under clothing. The crab louse is smaller and is found in pubic and underarm hair. Treatment is by insecticidal shampoo and clothing, towels, etc, that have been in contact must be washed in insecticidal soap and boil washed.

ITCH MITES (*Sarcoptes scabiei*)

A tiny animal which burrows into the skin producing a condition called scabies. It has eight legs and is around 0.3 mm long and 0.2 mm wide. The fertilised female burrows into the skin forming dark lines about 1 cm long. She lays around 60 eggs in the burrows which hatch in 4–8 days. The burrows are commonly seen between the fingers, on the front of the wrists, forearms or may be on male genitalia. They cause intense irritation, vesicles, papules and pustules. They are easily passed from person to person. Medical opinion should be sought and any clothing, towels, etc, that have come into contact with such a client must be burned.

FLEAS

The flea is an insect with three pairs of legs which enable it to jump long distances from host to host. It obtains nourishment by biting and sucking the blood of the host. The bites cause red spots usually found in groups; they are intensely itchy. Fleas lay eggs in dust, carpets or furniture. They can be eliminated by spraying with insecticides, washing clothing and bedding and thorough cleaning of soft furnishings. The flea was responsible for carrying the plague.

ENDOPARASITES

Figure 9.11   *Worms and flukes*

These include a variety of worms and flukes. Infestation is usually the result of poor standards of hygiene and insanitary conditions. Worms may be passed on to humans through contaminated food or water, while undercooked pork and beef are a source of tapeworms. Threadworms, tapeworms and roundworms live in the intestine and may cause diarrhoea, weakness and anaemia. Liver flukes live in the bile ducts and liver causing jaundice, while some serious types of fluke invade small blood vessels causing serious illness.

The body's defences are not effective against these infestations and drug treatment is essential to eliminate the worms. These anthelmintic drugs kill or paralyse the worms and they pass out of the body in faeces. If serious complications have occurred, other drugs may be necessary to deal with these.

Methods of controlling micro-organisms

The process of controlling micro-organisms in the salon is the responsibility of all therapists and must be taken seriously. Correct hygiene procedures must be adopted as a matter of routine. Instruments must always be cleaned after use and then sterilised or disinfected.

Various words are used to explain hygiene procedures. Their meaning must be clearly understood so that the appropriate methods are selected. Definitions are as follows:

- *Antibiotic.* An organic chemical substance which in dilute solution can destroy or inhibit the growth of bacteria and some other micro-organisms. They are used to treat infectious diseases in humans, animals and plants.

- *Antiseptic.* A chemical agent which destroys or inhibits the growth of micro-organisms on living tissues, thus limiting or preventing the harmful results of infection (usually used on wounds, sores or skin cleansing).
- *Aseptic methods.* Procedures adopted for creating conditions for avoiding infection.
- *Bactericide.* A chemical agent which, under defined conditions, is capable of killing bacteria, but not necessarily the spores.
- *Bacteriostat/fungistat.* Chemical agents which under defined conditions are capable of inhibiting the multiplication of bacteria/fungi.
- *Biocide, fungicide, virucide, sporicide.* These words imply the destruction of bacteria fungi, viruses and spores. Biocides kill everything.
- *Disinfectant.* A chemical agent which destroys micro-organisms but not spores (usually used on articles, implements, surfaces, drains, etc).
- *Sanitation.* The establishment of conditions favourable to health and preventing the spread of disease.
- *Sepsis/septic.* Being infected by bacteria; usually associated with pus formation.
- *Sterilisation.* The total destruction or removal of all living micro-organisms and their spores.

STERILISATION AND DISINFECTION

While it is impossible to create a perfectly sterile environment in the salon, every effort must be made to limit the growth and to destroy micro-organisms by practising high standards of hygiene. The clients and therapists must be protected from cross-infection.

Most treatments require the therapist to touch the client, therefore every precaution must be taken to prevent cross infection from one to the other.

The therapist's hands must be washed using bactericidal lotions and the client's skin must be cleaned by taking a shower or cleansing and toning the face for facial work and wiping over the area with surgical spirit for body treatments. Any small cuts and abrasions on the therapist's hands or on the client's skin must be covered with waterproof plaster. If there is any danger of blood seepage, the treatment should not be carried out.

For some treatments good quality fine surgical gloves could be worn to protect against any contamination. Care must be taken when removing gloves, peel carefully from the open wrist end so that the glove ends up inside out thus containing any contamination.

Extreme care must be taken when practising procedures which pierce the skin. In certain procedures, such as epilation, red vein therapy, etc, it is necessary to pierce the skin, but other procedures may result in blood loss due to accidental piercing of the skin. All blood spills must be dealt with immediately because serious diseases such as HIV and hepatitis can be transmitted via blood contamination. (see page 218).

Disposable needles must be used for treating clients in the salon; a new needle must be used at the commencement of treatment and disposed of after use. They should be carefully removed from the chuck using forceps and placed in a 'sharp's box'. Disposable equipment should always be used if it is economically viable. Reusable equipment should be sterilised if suitable otherwise must be disinfected.

Note: All equipment and instruments contaminated with blood or body fluids must be sterilised or disposed of in sealed plastic containers and incinerated.

CLEANING OF EQUIPMENT

All articles must be thoroughly clean before being sterilised or disinfected. The articles should be thoroughly soaked, washed and scrubbed with a hard brush in water and detergent. Care must be taken to reach the more inaccessible parts so that all matter is removed. Finally, they should be rinsed thoroughly under running water.

This procedure is very important for the following reasons:

1 To remove dirt and all organic matter which may be left on the article.
2 To remove all infective matter.
3 To remove all grease or oil which form a barrier and interfere with the sterilising or disinfecting process, reducing its effectiveness.
4 To remove all dirt and organic matter which would harden, forming a permanent coating on the articles. This would interfere with sterilising or disinfecting and would cause deterioration of certain instruments.

STERILISATION

Sterilisation is the best procedure for small instruments and should be a major consideration when purchasing these articles.

The therapist should check with the manufacturer that the materials are suitable for the chosen method of sterilisation. Instruments made of stainless steel and certain plastics are suitable, although sharp edges may be blunted by exposure to heat.

There are three main methods of sterilisation available, but they are not all suitable for use in the salon.

STERILISATION BY RADIATION

Two types of rays are used:
1 *Gamma radiation* is only suitable for use on a large scale. Articles to be sterilised are prepacked and exposed to radiation. Colour change indicators are used in the packages to show that sterlisation has been achieved. There is little temperature rise and it is, therefore, particularly useful for heat sensitive materials. Disposable needles are usually sterilised in this way. It has the advantage that materials can be prepacked before sterilisation.
2 *Ultraviolet radiation* is no longer recommended for sterilisation. It will destroy bacteria, but spores are resistant. It is also difficult to ensure penetration of the rays and articles require turning to ensure irradiation of all surfaces. Ultraviolet cabinets are frequently found in hair and beauty salons, and although they must not be used as sterilisers they can be used for storing articles after they have been sterilised.

Figure 9.12   *Ultraviolet cabinet. This will not sterilise but may be used for storage*

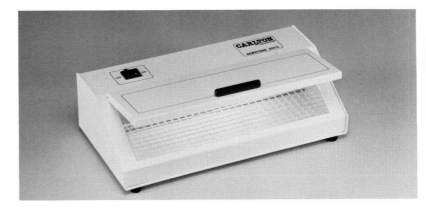

STERILISATION BY GASES

Two gases are used:

1 Ethylene oxide at a temperature of 20–56°C.
2 Formaldehyde at a temperature of 70°C.

These gases are used in chambers into which the articles are placed for a certain period of time. They are not suitable for salon use as they are difficult to handle and can form explosive mixtures with air. However, formaldehyde cabinets are still found in some salons.

STERILISATION BY HEAT (SUITABLE FOR USE IN SALONS)

Two methods can be used:

1 Dry heat.

2 Moist heat.

With all methods of heat sterilisation, the combination of correct temperature and time of exposure are necessary for sterility to be achieved. For moist heat, the pressure in the steriliser is also important. The sterilisation process can be broken up into four time factors:

1 Heating up time: the time taken for the steriliser to reach the sterilising temperature.
2 Heat penetration time: the time taken for all parts of the load to reach the sterilising temperature.
3 Holding time: this is the time required to sterilise the load at the selected temperture.
4 Safety time: this is an addition of 50 per cent to the holding time to ensure that resistant spores are destroyed.

Both methods are suitable for salon use as small models are manufactured for sterilising small instruments. Hot air ovens and glass bead sterilisers are used for dry heat sterilisation, while pressure vessels called autoclaves are used for moist heat.

The process of boiling in water is no longer considered as a method of sterilisation as spores will survive at this temperature. It is now considered to be a process of disinfecting.

Dry heat

Dry heat ovens. These ovens are electrically heated with a fan to circulate the air. A dial thermometer is fitted to indicate the temperature reached within the oven. Dry heat must reach a temperature of 140°C to kill bacterial spores. However, the higher the temperature, the shorter the exposure time. Therefore, temperatures of 150–180°C are commonly used. The following temperatures and corresponding timings are issued by the Medical Council:

Table J *Dry heat temperatures and timings*

Temperature 0°C	Exposure time in minutes
160	45
170	18
180	$7\frac{1}{2}$
190	$1\frac{1}{2}$

This covers both holding time and safety time.

Figure 9.13   *A glass bead steriliser*

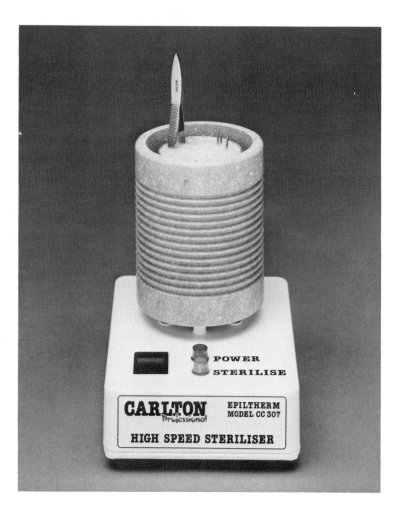

Glass bead sterilisers. These are suitable for very small articles (read the manufacturer's instructions). They are made of an electrically heated box covered by an insulating case. The box is filled with tiny glass beads. The temperature can range from 190–300°C, and the sterilising times will vary accordingly; be sure to follow the instructions on the model.

These have the disadvantages that they are only suitable for small objects, eg needles or forceps, and that the objects cannot be fully immersed. Therefore, a small part outside the beads will remain unsterilised.

MOIST HEAT

Figure 9.14   *An automatic electronic autoclave*

Autoclave. This is a vessel which boils water under pressure so that higher temperatures can be reached. It sterilises by steam under pressure. Water boils at atmospheric pressure at 100°C, but if the pressure is increased, then the temperature at which the water boils is raised. The autoclave is a closed vessel which is constructed to withstand high pressure so that the temperature of the water and steam will reach the 100–150°C needed for sterilisation. Air must be eliminated from the vessel in order to achieve the following pressure/temperature relationships.

Table K *Pressure temperature relationships for the autoclave*

Pressure in psi (pounds per square inch)	Boiling point °C
10	115
15	121
32	134

For sterilsing with moist heat, the following temperatures and corresponding timings are issued by the Medical Research Council:

Table L *Temperatures and timings for sterilising with moist heat*

Temperature °C	Timing in minutes
121	15
126	10
134	3

This covers both holding and safety times.

Very large autoclaves are manufactured for commercial and hospital use. For salon use, smaller, simple automatic autoclaves are now manufactured for small-scale sterilisation. The required volume of water is placed in the steriliser. Articles to be sterilised are placed in dishes or on racks within the autoclave. The items must be loaded with care to avoid trapping large bubbles of air, which could interfere with pressure, temperature and timing relationships. Small dishes and vessels should be placed on their side and not inverted. Instruments should be positioned so that steam can contact all surfaces; they should not be placed in bundles. Once the steriliser is switched on, the cycle is automatically controlled.

Cleaned articles can be loaded at the end of the day and the steriliser switched on and left to complete its cycle, then unloaded the following morning. Colour change indicators are available to ensure that sterilising conditions have been reached.

DISINFECTANTS

Equipment made from materials which are not suitable for sterilisation must be disinfected. Also shelves, work surfaces and other surfaces should be regularly wiped over with disinfectant solutions.

A wide variety of products are available, and any information regarding the products should be carefully studied in order to make an informed choice.

Disinfectants must be used in the concentrations and timings recommended; if they are further diluted their effectiveness is reduced. Most disinfectants are more effective at higher temperatures. Other factors which may reduce effectiveness are:

1 The presence of organic matter, such as dead skin, dried blood or vomit; as previously stated, all articles should be cleaned before disinfection.
2 Some disinfectants are inactivated by hard water, while others are inactivated by soaps.

3 Effectiveness is progressively diminished with age. Store only for the recommended time; do not use after expiry date.

Disinfectants, if incorrectly stored, used and diluted, can themselves become infected and be a source of infection.

EXAMPLES OF DISINFECTANTS

- Alcohols such as *methanol, ethanol, isopropanol.* They form the basis of methylated spirit and surgical spirit. Alcohol is most effective at 70 per cent strength, ie seven parts alcohol diluted by three parts water. Bactericidal in action, they kill bacteria but not spores, and their effect against viruses is limited.

  Uses: wiping down of all surfaces
  disinfecting electrodes, ventouse, etc
  surgical spirit swabs used on the skin

- Aldehydes such as *Formaldehyde* and *glutaraldehyde.* Formaldehyde gas is soluble in water and used as formalin. It is highly irritating to tissues and must not be applied to the skin. It is biocidal in action and will destory bacteria, viruses and fungi and some spores. It is only used in specialised industries.

  Glutaraldehyde is an extremely useful disinfectant known as *Cydex.* Germicidal in action, it will kill bacteria, viruses, fungi and most spores if used for a specified length of time. Immersion of over 10 hours would cover everything. It is highly irritating to eyes and skin, and rubber gloves and a surgical mask should be worn when handling this disinfectant.

  Uses: Cydex – immersion of instruments and other equipment
  for disinfection

- Diguanides, such as *chlorhexidine* (Hibitane). Another good disinfectant. It is less irritating to the skin and eyes than some other disinfectants, but can cause dryness. Effective against bacteria and fungi but less effective against viruses and spores.

  It is used with detergents in products such as *Hibiscrub,* or with alcohol in products such as *Dispray.*

  Uses: Hibiscrub – hand washing or skin cleansing
  Dispray – cleansing of surfaces

- Halogens such as *chlorine* and *iodine.* Chlorine is a very effective and cheap disinfectant. It is irritating to eyes and skin and must be used with care as directed. Wear rubber gloves.

  It is effective against bacteria some spore and viruses. It is corrosive and not suitable for use on metal instruments. Commercially available products are *Milton* and *Domestos.*

Uses: Milton – immersion of non-metal instruments, eg made of plastic or glass

Domestos – wiping of surfaces, floors, sinks, sanitary ware, etc; use as directed

Preparations containing *iodine* stain the skin brown. They are mainly used as skin disinfectants, but not in beauty therapy.

- Phenols such as *carbolic acid*. Carbolic acid was a very popular antiseptic in the past. It is found in products such as *Lysol* and *Izal*.

Uses: Izal – cleansing sanitary ware, drains

Dettol – used on skin

Dettinox – used to wipe down surfaces

- *Quaternary ammonium compounds*. These are bacteriostatic preventing the multiplication of micro-organisms. Used mainly with detergents for skin and wound cleansing. Found in products such as *Cetavlon* and *Savlon*.

Uses: cleansing of skin and wounds

Salon hygiene

This is the responsibility of all therapists and must be taken very seriously. As well as protecting the client, the therapist must protect herself.

Great care must be taken when handling unsterilised sharps and instruments to avoid cuts and stabs which may result in infection. Great care must also be taken when handling disinfectants. These are strong chemicals capable of destroying micro-organisms, but they can also cause damage to the handler, producing burns, etc. When handling these substances, rubber gloves and a surgical mask should always be worn and care taken not to splash the skin, eyes, nose, mouth. Any drops on these areas must be thoroughly rinsed off immediately with cold water.

The following are guidelines which should be followed for establishing high standards or practice and hygiene in the salon.

1 Disposable instruments and equipment should be used whenever possible.
2 Any instrument which pierces the skin should be disposed of and placed in a sharp's box. If this is not practical, then the instrument must be sterilised.
3 All metal instruments should be washed and sterilised if suitable using one of the following methods:
   (a) Dry heat bead sterilisation – this is useful for needles, forceps and other small instruments. However, it is

important to remember that any part of the instrument which is not immersed remains unsterilised.

(b) By autoclave – moist heat under pressure – this is the best method for all articles made of suitable materials. Metal instruments not suitable for the autoclave must be disinfected in a product which does not cause rusting.

4 All articles that are unsuitable for sterilisation must be washed and disinfected. Immerse for the directed time in products such as Cydex, Milton or Barbicide.

5 Articles made from other materials should be cleaned as follows:

Glass and perspex – Check with manufacturers if the items are suitable for autoclaving as the heat may cause deterioration.

Vacuum suction cups – Wash thoroughly with water and detergent using a small brush to reach inaccessible parts, rinse, dry, then immerse for the stated time in Milton, Cydex and Barbicide.

High Frequency electrodes – Keep the metal connecting end dry. Carefully wipe the electrode face with water and detergent, rinse, dry, then wipe over with surgical spirit, wash again and dry.

Rubber pads – Keep the connecting end dry. Wash carefully with water and detergent, use a soft brush to remove any dirt, rinse and dry. Circles of wet lint or viscose placed between the skin and the electrode will prevent contamination and can be disposed of after treatment or thoroughly washed. Disinfectants can cause deterioration of the rubber and should not be used unless recommended by the manufacturer.

Viscose or foam pads – Soak and rinse in cold water to remove any chemicals then wash in hot water and detergent, rinse and dry.

6 The client's skin should be cleaned before treatment using surgical spirit or Savlon wipes. Any cuts must be covered with waterproof plasters.

7 Therapists should wash their hands before and after treatment using a product such as Hibiscrub. Dry with a disposable towel or hot air dryer.

8 Working surfaces should be wiped down frequently during the day using 70 per cent alcohol or products such as Dispray. At the end of each day, wash down with water and detergent and wipe over with 10 per cent Domestos. Chairs, stools, couches and trolleys should also be cleaned in this way at the end of the day.

9 A plentiful supply of good quality towels should be available for covering the couch and for client use. These should be boil washed after each client. Disposable paper sheets should be used to protect the couch cover.

10 Commodities should be chosen with care as creams and lotions, etc, in tubes or narrow necked bottles have a smaller surface to be contaminated than wide necked jars.

11 Always use a new clean spatula to remove creams or lotions; do not return any contaminated article back to the product. This is a particular problem when using or applying make up. Eye shadow, liner, lipstick, powder, etc, should be scraped or removed from the container and placed on a palette. Disposable sponges and cotton wool buds should then be used for applying make up from the palette. Clients can be encouraged to have their own set of make up, brushes, etc.

12 A first-aid box should be positioned in an obvious easily accessible place.

13 The stock cupboard should be clean neat and tidy. Commodities should be clearly labelled showing the use – by date, which should not be exceeded.

14 Bins with plastic liners should be easily reached. All waste should be immediately disposed of; wet waste should first be wrapped in paper. The waste bins should be emptied and disinfected every night and clean liners inserted.

A special sharp's box should be available for disposal of needles, razors, etc, which could penetrate the skin. Special arrangement for collection and subsequent disposal of these boxes can be organised by contacting the local environmental health officer.

15 Toilet facilities should be easily accessible. These should be well ventilated and disinfected at least once a day. Sanitary ware and floors can be cleaned using Domestos solution.

16 Blood spills must be dealt with immediately. Wear rubber gloves. Pour on neat chlorine, eg Domestos, leave for 10 minutes then wipe off with a disposable cloth. Wash with water and detergent and wipe over with more Domestos.

Personal hygiene

1 A daily bath or shower will maintain cleanliness of the skin and remove stale sweat, dirt and grease.

2 The use of an antiperspirant after bathing will prevent excessive sweating and the odour of stale sweat.

3 Underwear and tights should be changed daily and washed thoroughly in soapy water, as they absorb body odours.

4 White shortsleeved overalls should be crisp and well laundered. A clean overall should be worn every other day. Therapists should not wear the uniform out of doors. Outdoor clothing should be changed in a cloakroom to prevent micro-organisms being brought into the salon.

5 Hair must be clean and worn short or tied off the face.

6 The teeth must be cleaned regularly – twice a day; a mouth wash can be used after eating. Smoking or spicy foods should be avoided. Regular dental checks are necessary to prevent the build up of plaque.

7 Hands should receive particular care. They should be washed frequently before and after treatments, after handling any contaminated equipment or using the toilet. A bactericidal soap should be used. A good hand cream should be applied nightly to keep the skin soft and in good condition. Always wear rubber gloves when dealing with blood spills or disinfectants.

8 Nails should be kept short, well manicured and spotlessly clean; organisms can be harboured under the nail. Any nail enamel should be subtle and immaculate – well buffed nails look more natural and any dirt under the nail plate can be quickly seen and removed.

9 Feet should be well cared for. They should be washed and dried thoroughly at least once a day. Talc or foot powder should be used. Nails must be cut regularly straight across. Well fitting flat shoes without holes and peeptoes will protect the feet and avoid pressure points.

10 Therapists with colds or any throat infections should not treat clients if possible, but the wearing of a surgical mask will greatly reduce the likelihood of cross-infection. Any cuts or infections of the hands or nails should be treated and covered with finger stalls; large areas of infection mean that the therapist should not be working.

11 Food and drink should not be consumed nor stored in the salon working area. Contamination could be transferred to the food and then to the mouth.

Setting up a salon

The establishment of a hygienic, healthy environment is of prime importance to anyone setting up a salon. Consideration should be given to the following:

1 Rooms should be light, warm and well ventilated.

2 The walls should be covered with a material which can be frequently cleaned and washed down.

3 The floors should be hard, washable surfaces, such as vinyl.

4 Curtains or hanging should be of fabrics that are easy to wash and care for.

5 Couches, chairs, stools, etc, should be covered with smooth, washable materials, such as vinyl or plastic, and kept in good repair.

6 Trolleys, shelves and worktops should be of hard, smooth surfaces, free of cracks and easy to clean. They should be kept neat and tidy and uncluttered.

7 There must be handbasins or sinks with a hot water supply so that therapists can wash their hands between treating clients. Hot air dryers or disposable towels should be available for drying.

A shower should be available for clients to use if required before treatment. All these washing facilities must be kept scrupulously clean.

8 An autoclave should be available for sterilising instruments.

9 An easily accessible stock cupboard should store clearly labelled commodites.

10 A first-aid box must be placed in an obvious easily accessible position.

11 A bin with plastic liner should be available in each working area.

12 A plentiful supply of towels should be available. They should be of good quality as they are boil washed after each client.

13 A sharp's box must be available and arrangements made for its collection.

14 Good quality products should be used. Those in tubes or ampules are less likely to become contaminated than those in wide-necked jars.

15 Toilet facilities should be easily accessible and kept scrupulously clean.

16 A small cloakroom or large cupboard should be available for hanging outdoor clothes.

SUMMARY

- If micro-organisms invade the body in sufficient numbers to overcome the immune system, they will cause disease.
- Micro-organisms which infect the body are bacteria, viruses, fungi or yeasts and protozoa.

IMMUNITY

- Natural immunity is acquired by previous contact with a disease, the antibodies remain in the body or acquired via the placenta or milk from the mother.
- Artificial immunity is acquired from vaccines introduced into the body, which stimulate the immune system to produce antibodies, or may be acquired by the transfer of antibodies from a person who has recovered from the disease.

- Bacteria, single cell organisms, non-pathogenic or pathogenic – cocci, bacilli, spirochetes; diseases – boils, impetigo, sore throat, meningitis, pneumonia, typhoid fever, syphilis, cholera.
- Viruses: multiply and destroy the host cells; diseases – colds, influenza, poliomyelitis, mumps, chicken pox, herpes simplex and zoster, warts, hepatitis, HIV.
- Hepatitis and HIV are found in semen, saliva and blood.
- Ways of transmitting a virus: through blood transfusion, drug users sharing needles, the transfer of blood from an infected person into a cut or puncture of the skin, infected women can pass it to the foetus.
- Fungi: yeasts and moulds; diseases – tinea of various parts of body, thrush, fungal infections of organs such as heart and lungs.
- Protozoa: single-celled animals; diseases – sleeping sickness, malaria, amoebic dysentery.
- Parasites live in or on another living organism.

  1 Ectoparasites live outside host, eg lice and fleas.
  2 Endoparasites live inside host, eg worms and flukes.

- Sterilisation is the total destruction of microbes and spores.
- Methods of sterilisation in a beauty salon:

  1 Bead steriliser – small articles only.
  2 Autoclave.

- Disinfecting: the use of a chemical agent which destroys microbes but not spores.
- Disinfectants for use in a salon:
  70% alcohol: methylated spirit and surgical spirit
  isopropyl alcohol
  Glutaraldehyde: Cydex
  Chlorine: Milton, Domestos
  Phenols: Dettol, Dettinox, Izal, Lysol
  Ammonium compounds: Cetavlon, Savlon
  Diquamides: Hibitane, Hibiscrub, Dispray
- Suggested uses:
  For soaking and immersion of implements: Cydex, Milton and Barbicide
  Wiping VS cups and electrodes: surgical spirit, isopropyl, alcohol, Salon wipes
  Cleaning surfaces: Dettinox, Dispray, Domestos
  Cleaning skin: surgical spirit, Savlon
  Washing hands: Hibiscrub and other bactericidal soaps
  Toilets and sanitary ware: Dettol, Izal, Domestos.

QUESTIONS

1 Define the terms 'infection' and 'infestation'.
2 Explain the differences between bacteria and viruses.
3 Give three diseases caused by each of the following:
   (a) bacteria;
   (b) viruses;
   (c) fungi;
   (d) protozoa.
4 Explain the term 'natural immunity'.
5 Give two methods of producing artificial immunity.
6 List the ways in which microbes may enter the body.
7 Explain how microbes may be transmitted.
8 List the forms of the hepatitis virus.
9 Explain how the hepatitis B virus and HIV may be transmitted.
10 Define the terms 'ectoparasite' and 'endoparasite' and give three examples of each.

11 Define the following:
   (a) sterilisation;
   (b) sanitation;
   (c) disinfectant;
   (d) antiseptic;
   (e) bactericide;
   (f) Biocide.
12 Identify which of the following are methods of sterilisation:
   (a) Immersion in Milton.
   (b) Glass bead boxes.
   (c) Ultraviolet cabinets.
   (d) Immersion in Cidex.
   (e) Autoclaving.
13 Explain how you would deal with the following equipment after use:
   (a) Epilation needles.
   (b) Cuticle knives.
   (c) Vacuum suction cups.
   (d) Forceps.
14 List ten factors to be considered for maintaining high standards of salon hygiene.

Glossary of terms

Blood pressure. The pressure exerted against the artery walls, during contraction of the heart – systolic pressure; and relaxation of the heart – diastolic pressure. Normal BP is around 120 (systolic)/80 (diastolic).

Connector or inter-neurones. These connect one neurone with another.

Couperosed skin. A redness of the skin.

Desquamation. A flaking or erosion of the surface layer of the statum corneum of the skin.

Diaphorectic effect. An increase in the production of sweat.

Electrolyte. A chemical compound which dissociates into ions and carries a current.

Erythema. A redenning of the skin; this happens as a result of vasodilation.

Heart rate. The rate at which the heart beats; this is the same as the pulse rate.

Hyperaemia. An increase in blood flow to an area.

Metabolic rate. The rate of chemical reaction in body cells.

Metabolites. Waste products of metabolism.

Motor nerves or neurones. These nerves transmit impulses from brain and spinal cord to muscles and glands.

Occlude. To stop or obstruct.

Oedema or edima. Swelling of an area due to excess fluid.

Phlebitis. Inflammation of a vein.

Sebaceous glands. Glands in the skin which secrete a fatty substance called sebum.

Seborrhoea. Excessive secretion of sebum from sebaceous glands.

Sensory nerves or neurones. These nerves transmit impulses from sensory organs, such as skin, eyes and ears, to the spinal cord and brain.

Stasis. An area of stagnation due to poor circulation.

Telangiectasis. Small, red spots on the skin caused by dilated capillaries.

Tension nodules. Areas within a muscle where muscle fibres show increase in tone.

Thrombosis. The formation of a blood clot in blood vessels.

Vasoconstriction. Constriction of blood vessels, i.e. the lumen get smaller.

Vasodilation. Dilation of blood vessels, i.e. the lumen of the blood vessels get larger.

Bibliography

Bennett, Ruth, *The Science of Beauty Therapy* (Hodder & Stoughton, 1992).

Gray, H., *Gray's Anatomy* (Churchill Livingston, 1980).

Freemantle, Michael, *Chemistry in Action* (McMillan Ed. Std, 1987).

Foster and Palastanga, *Clayton's Electrotherapy* (Bailliere Tindall, 1987).

Hutchinson Encyclopedia (Guild Publishing London, 1988).

Kahn, Joseph, *Principles and Practice of Electrotherapy* (Churchill Livingston, 1987).

Peberdy, W. G., *Sterilisation and Hygiene in the Beauty Professions* (1987).

Ross, J. S. and Wilson K. J. W., *Anatomy and Physiology* (Churchill Livingston, 1988).

Simmons, John *The Beauty Salon and its Equipment* (McMillan, 1989)

Index